Other books by Jonathan Robinson

The Little Book of Big Questions
200 Ways to Explore Your Spiritual Nature

Communication Miracles for Couples
Easy and Effective Tools to Create More Love and Less Conflict

Shortcuts to Bliss
The 50 Best Ways to Improve Relationships, Connect with Spirit, and make Dreams Come True

Shortcuts to Success

Shortcuts to
Success

The Absolute Best Ways to Master Your
Time, Health, Relationships, and Finances

Jonathan Robinson

CONARI PRESS
Berkeley, California

Copyright © 2000 by Jonathan Robinson

All Rights Reserved. No part of this book may be used or reproduced in any manner whatsoever without written permission, except in the case of brief quotations in critical articles or reviews. For information, contact: Conari Press, 2550 Ninth Street, Suite 101, Berkeley, CA 94710-2551.

Conari Press books are distributed by Publishers Group West

Cover Illustration: Kurt Vargo
Interior Illustrations: Copyright © Ashleigh Brilliant, Santa Barbara, CA. www.ashleighbrilliant.com
Reprinted by permission.

Library of Congress Cataloging-in-Publication Data

Robinson, Jonathan, 1942–
Shortcuts to success : the absolute best ways to master your time, health,
relationships, and finances / Jonathan Robinson.
p.   cm.
ISBN 1-57324-188-1 (trade pbk.)
1. Success—Psychological aspects. I. Title.

BF637.S8R63 2000
646.7—dc21   99-042066

Printed in the United States of America on recycled paper.

00 01 02 03   Data Repro   10 9 8 7 6 5 4 3 2 1

Shortcuts to Success

LIFE IS THE ONLY GAME

IN WHICH THE OBJECT OF THE GAME

IS TO LEARN THE RULES.

Ashleigh Brilliant

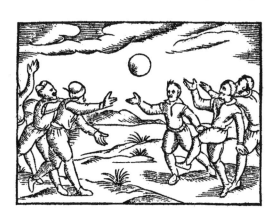

Getting Started

We live in an era of constant change. In order to create a high quality of life when so much activity is continually happening, it's more important than ever to master certain skills. The methods presented in this book to help you master your time, health, relationships, and finances are some of the finest tools available for "building" success. They can help you manifest the life you desire more quickly, easily, and effectively than you may have ever thought possible. Don't underestimate their power. Even just a single idea or method presented in this book can have a profound impact on the quality of your life.

Webster's dictionary defines "success" as "the achievement of something desired." However, in our materialistic culture, "success" has often been confused with fame and fortune. There is nothing wrong with riches and respect, but true success is more than just that. In order to feel successful, we need to have various aspects of our lives in balance. Millions of dollars will do you little good if your health is poor, people dislike you, and your life feels out of control. On the other hand, avoiding the area of finances can lead to a life of constant anxiety about money. If you can learn the shortcuts to creating good health, relationships, time for what you enjoy, and financial prosperity, then you'll likely feel successful. This book will help you learn about some of the most efficient, effective, and practical ways to create the life you really want.

I TRY TO TAKE
ONE DAY AT A TIME,

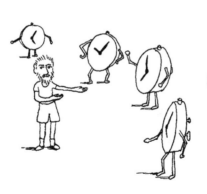

BUT SOMETIMES
SEVERAL DAYS
ATTACK ME
AT ONCE.

Ashleigh Brilliant

Mastering Your Time

For most Westerners, poverty has taken on a new meaning. Instead of feeling a lack of money, a majority of people are feeling a lack of time. Indeed, we do have plenty of material prosperity. Even middle-class folks of today live better than kings lived just fifty years ago! Our civilization gives us the riches of libraries, endless channels of free entertainment to watch, telephones, supermarkets, and air conditioned cars to speed us wherever we want to go. Yet we don't necessarily have the *time* to enjoy all our good fortune. Unlike fifty years ago, people spend a lot of their lives rushing around, feeling like they lack the time to do the things they truly desire. To a large extent, we've traded our precious time for more money and the many comforts it can buy. However, for those who feel an ongoing poverty of time, there is hope. As you learn about and use the time management ideas in this section, you'll feel like you're in control of your time—rather than it being in control of you.

I assume that if you're reading this book, you're already familiar with some basic time management ideas. Nevertheless, I hope to introduce you to several ideas you may not have heard before. While some of these ideas may not fit your current lifestyle, even one new idea taken from the following chapters can significantly impact your entire destiny. After all, time is more than money. The manner in which you use your time determines the quality and direction of your life. Fortunately, time management is a skill that is easily learned. As you use the ideas in this section, you will feel like you are accomplishing more with your time, and using it to experience greater personal satisfaction.

1. Know Your Unique Path to Success

The Three Keys to Being On Target

In order to be successful, you first need to define what success means to you. While Western culture may define success in terms of riches, fame, beauty, and youth, these things may not be what *you* really want. I first learned the importance of defining what I was after when I was in college. My roommate, Tony, was a varsity basketball player who was always challenging me to a game of one-on-one basketball. At first, I avoided the challenge, but finally I caved in. I said, "I'll play you a game on one condition: I get to bring any one-ounce gadget onto the court and place it wherever I want. Tony agreed. We went to the court and I brought out my one ounce "gadget"—which was a blindfold, and I strategically placed it over Tony's eyes. Then I said, "Let the games begin!" Admittedly, the game still ended up being rather close. Yet, because I knew exactly what I was aiming for—and Tony didn't—I beat him despite my complete lack of skill. Knowing what you're aiming for is more important than luck, skill, or expertise.

In order to define what success is to you, it can be helpful to think about when you've felt the happiest in your past. When were three times in your life that you were, for a period of at least a month, rather happy and excited about your life? If you can, write a very brief description of these three times. As you review these three times in your life, do you notice any similar themes or events that occurred during each of these times? For example, were you traveling during these times, or were you moving forward in your career? Perhaps on each of these occasions you were in a rewarding relationship, or you were enjoying a leisurely pace of life. Whatever you notice about these periods in your life, take note. If they brought you a feeling of satisfaction in the past, they could likely bring you a similar feeling in the future. Therefore, if traveling made you happy in the past, you would likely feel successful if you could travel more in the future. Simple.

Unfortunately, it's easy to fall into *other* people's view of success and lose our own. When I was in junior high school, I fell into my mom's dream for me to do very well in school. In the school I was in, if you got straight A's for a full year, you got a little pin from the principal. Well, I worked real hard to live up to my mother's good intentions for me on how she defined success. By foregoing my social life, I managed to get straight A's for a full year. A couple of years ago while cleaning out some drawers, I found the cheap, gold-plated pin I received for achieving straight A's. I looked at that $2 pin and realized that this was the booby prize for going after someone else's idea of success. Don't let that happen to you. Instead, remember what has really made you happy in the past, and aim for that in the future.

A second way to be on target toward your own criteria for success is to figure out what you would do if you had a million dollars in the bank. What would you spend it on? Choose three or four things. Let's say you'd buy a house, purchase a nice car, give some money away to environmental causes, and keep a fair share in the bank. For each thing you'd spend money on, ask yourself, "What *feeling* might I get from spending money on that item?" For instance, if you'd buy a house, you could ask, "What feeling would I hope to get from owning my own home?" Perhaps the answer would be "I'd have more security and peace of mind." Then ask, "Why would I want to give money away to environmental causes?" Your answer to that might be, "To have a feeling of contributing to the greater good."

Once you know what you'd spend money on, and the underlying feelings you'd hope to experience from those purchases, you have some powerful information. The reason people want money is because they think they'll be able to convert their money into the emotional experiences they most desire. By making a list of what you'd want to spend extra money on, you can come to realize what emotional experiences you *most* desire in life. For instance, if you realize that you want a house, money in the bank, and a cruise vacation because you think they'll all bring you more peace, then you'd be smart to focus on having more peace in your life. The more peace you have, the more likely you'll feel successful. On the other hand, the less peace—or the more busy you are—the less likely you'll feel successful. Since we all crave different feelings, it's important to know what are the specific feelings that are most important to you.

We all want to have a lot of positive feelings in our life. Yet, not all positive feelings are created equal. Some people will do or pay anything for a moment of adventure, whereas others will avoid adventure at all cost. In the previous exercise of figuring out what you'd do with a million extra dollars, you got to see that certain feelings are more important to you than others. Another way to define success for yourself is to simply rate different experiences on a hierarchy. Below are ten different things most people want. Try rating them from one to ten, with one being the most important, and ten being the least important.

_____Comfort	_____Achievement
_____Inner Peace	_____Prestige/Respect
_____Security	_____Power
_____Intimacy	_____Friendship
_____Spiritual Growth	_____Freedom

This is a difficult exercise to do. After all, it's hard to choose whether "intimacy" is more important than "inner peace," or any of the other choices you have to make in this exercise. Yet, we unconsciously make decisions all the time about our priorities that determine our future. By consciously knowing what you most value, you're in a better position to determine how to spend your time in a way that is likely to maximize your level of success. For example, if you value "friendship" above all else, but you spend most of your time pursuing security, achievement, and power, then your life will feel stressful and unfulfilling. On the other hand, if you spend most of your time pursuing the values that are truly meaningful to you, then you'll likely feel good about your life.

Success means different things to different people. By defining success in terms of your values, your previous periods of happiness, and the emotions you most desire, you can better know what to aim for in the future. The more you can define your unique version of success, the more likely you'll be able to achieve it.

2. Get More Done In Less Time

The Power Tools of Time Management

If you want to build a house, having an electric saw is infinitely better than using a hand-held saw. Some tools are simply much more effective than others. When trying to make efficient use of your time, there are proven "power tools" that have been shown to make a major difference in how much a person can get done. After surveying various books on time management, and trying various methods in my own life, I realized that five specific tools are the most effective in being able to accomplish more in less time. Although you may be familiar with some or all of these methods, familiarity isn't enough. You need to be as committed to them as you are to brushing your teeth each day. Since we live in the busiest culture in the history of humanity, knowing how to get control of one's time is no longer just a "nice idea," it's a necessity. These tools will help you survive, psychologically and financially, in this crazy time we live in.

1) Prioritize! Studies show that, for every minute spent prioritizing, five minutes are saved. That means you're getting a 500 percent return on your time investment. Not bad. You probably know of various ways to prioritize your day. Listing all the things you might do on a given day and then ranking them in their order of importance can be helpful. The most important aspect of prioritizing your day is *doing it each and every day.* Many people who know of the benefits of prioritization still fail to do it. If you're one of these people, then learn to reward yourself immediately after you prioritize your day. In my case, I eat breakfast immediately following making my daily "to do" list and ranking the order of which I'll do things. Since I love eating breakfast, the list always gets done.

2) Delegate. How do you think CEOs and presidents are able to give speeches around the country, make hundreds of decisions, keep up on their phone calls and mail, and still have time to play so much golf? They delegate. They make a distinction between things that *only* they can do, and things that other people can do. They don't write their own speeches, they don't read their own mail, they barely play their own golf. The sad truth is that you can't be extremely successful unless you learn to delegate effectively—because there is only so much one person can do. Delegating can be scary. High achievers are used to being in control, and delegating is a process of giving up control. However, as you practice delegating, you come to

realize that there are some people you can trust to get a job done, and some you can't. Therefore, like any skill, it gets easier over time since you soon learn who you can count on.

3) Learn to say no. This has always been difficult for me. In an attempt to be a nice guy, I have always tried to be all things for all people. After years of doing this, I'm finally seeing the necessity of telling people, "I understand your need, but I'm sorry, I just don't have the available time to help you." I've memorized that sentence and try to say it whenever someone approaches me for a favor that I don't feel passionate about, or would require more than just a minute of my time. If you have a difficult time doing this, your life will soon become crazy. I now have a note card by my phone that says the word "NO!" in big letters. Several times a day people call me up and ask for my time—free of charge. Whereas I used to say "Yes" to almost all of them, now I say "No" to about 80 percent of them. It's amazing how much more time this one simple technique has given me to do what I consider most important.

4) Learn to ask the simple question, "Considering my long-term goals and objective, what's the best use of my time right now?" Just asking this question throughout the day will help focus your mind in beneficial ways. Normally, we are subconsciously asking ourselves a different question, such as some variation on "What do I have to do next?" That question can lead people to focus on short-term, inconsequential items, rather than on more important, long-term goals. As you think in a broader sense about the best use of your time, you may see things that were invisible to you before. In addition, you may start to avoid certain time wasters, such as unnecessary meetings, phone calls, and paper work.

5) Learn the 80/20 rule. Basically, this rule states that 20 percent of your time creates 80 percent of what you accomplish. The challenge is to always focus on the key behaviors that are the best use of your time. The 80/20 rule also applies to the people you deal with. In this context it could be said that 20 percent of your customers will account for 80 percent of your business. Once again, the challenge is to isolate the 20 percent who are the most productive to work with, and focus on them. As you begin to look at your customers, your time, and your daily activities through the concept of the 80/20 rule, you'll start to see that some things are better left undone as you focus on the people and activities that create results.

In applying the 80/20 rule in my own life, I recently discovered that I was spending a lot of time preparing for and teaching a class at the local city college—which netted very little money. On the other hand, I used to spend very little time marketing myself to various organizations as a professional speaker. Despite spending just a couple of hours a week marketing myself in this way, I discovered that about a third of my income came from such talks during the previous year. Therefore, this year I have begun to devote more time to marketing myself as a speaker. So far, this better "investment" in my time is paying off very well.

Which of these tools are you failing to make use of on a consistent basis? Make a commitment to yourself to practice the ones that you have been hesitant to use. While practicing new habits can be difficult at first, you'll soon notice that you seem to magically have more time.

3. Take As Many Vacations as You Want

The Vacation Commitment Experiment

One day I called my friend, Susan, and asked her how she was. She said, "Things are great. Joe and I just got back from another week-long vacation." I realized that, just about every time I talked to Susan, she had recently gone on vacation. I was a bit annoyed and jealous. "How do you take so many vacations?" I asked. Her reply made me even more annoyed, "We simply make it a priority." I felt a certain amount of self-pity as I shot back, "Boy, I wish my life was set up so I could take so much time off." In a compassionate, yet direct manner, Susan replied, "You can if it's important enough to you. Joe and I just decided we'd take eight weeks off each year. There's a lot of resistance to doing that, but we're committed to living the life that we want to live."

I hung up the phone practically enraged, thinking, "Yeah, but I've got bills to pay, work to do. I could never do that." Then a lightbulb in my brain went off. I heard the still, small voice inside my head say, "The only thing stopping you is fear. You could take eight weeks off a year if you really wanted to." I knew that voice was right. So I decided to give it a trial run for six months. I vowed I would take off four weeks in the next six months as an experiment. If my life and finances fell apart as a result, I would never do it again. If it worked, then maybe, just maybe, I would do it for another six months. So began my vacation commitment experiment.

We all have plenty of reasons why we can't possibly do the things we really want to do in life. Mortgages, kids, stressful jobs—the list is endless. However, where there's a will, there's a way. In 1991, I decided that I wanted to take six months off to travel around the world. At the time I had no money and a job I was locked into. Since it was obvious I couldn't go without any money, I made the commitment to leave in a year. It's amazing how things fall in line when you have a clearly stated goal and you announce it to the world. As I proclaimed my intentions, other people helped me get excited about my trip. Soon, there was a momentum of money being saved, an itinerary being set, and plans to tighten up various loose ends in my life. That trip ended up being the best six months of my life.

What are your vacation dreams? Do you want to travel around the world, or simply take mini-vacations on a more regular basis? I suggest you make a specific commitment as to how much time you'd like to take off this next year. I have found that my vacations not only add to the quality of my life, but also help me manifest more effectively in my career. Many of my best ideas have been born along a lonely stretch of beach or a winding forest path. Time off from the stresses of modern-day life helps to rejuvenate your soul and clarify the directions you want to go in life. It won't happen unless you commit to a specific, doable plan.

There are no rules as to what you should commit to. In order to come up with a plan that's right for you, however, it can be helpful to consider the following three questions:

1. Does a long vacation or several short vacations better fit in with my lifestyle, desires, and needs?

2. How much time off have I taken in recent years, and might I benefit from trying to take a little more time away from work?

3. Based on the answers to the two previous questions, what would be a reasonable plan I could commit to regarding time away from work over the course of the next year?

Every year I ask myself these three questions, and come up with a new plan. This past year, I decided to take five weeks off in a row, along with four mini-vacations of five days each. The key to success is to schedule your vacation time far off in the future (otherwise the time will get eaten up), and then stick with this commitment just as if it were a contract with an employer. Once you've made and scheduled your vacations, tell the appropriate people in your life (family, employer, etc.) so they have time to adjust to your schedule. In some cases, you may have to change your commitment to meet their needs, but do your best to hold on to your vacation dreams.

In the United States, people are typically given only two weeks of paid vacation time. Yet in many European countries five to eight weeks a year is standard. Nobody on their deathbed has said, "I wish I had spent more time at the office or watching TV." I know that making such a commitment can be scary, that's why I suggest you start off easy. Once you see that the world doesn't end as soon as you turn off your cellular phone, you'll be emboldened to keep going.

Since so many people are addicted to work, it can be helpful to add a certain punch to your commitment. You might try buying the plane tickets to your destination, even if the trip is several months away. You can also begin informing your employer, customers, or family of times you won't be available. You can make a deal with yourself that if you don't take the time off that you plan, you'll penalize yourself in some manner. For example, I now state that if I fail to keep any of my vacation plans, I will pay for the hotel I'm not using as a penalty for not going. Since I am somewhat cheap, this penalty has worked. Only once in the last three years have I missed the trip I had planned—and therefore paid the price. I'm not likely to waste money like that again anytime soon.

4. How to Do What's Most Important to You

The Art of Prioritizing Your Life

When people say they don't "have enough time," what they're really saying is they feel they are not spending as much time as they would like doing what's truly important to them. Since time is a limited resource, the best way to solve this problem is to clarify what *is* most important, and eliminate or delegate what is of lesser significance. To aid in this process, I've found five little-used life management tools to be very helpful:

- In order to know what's most important to you, it's helpful to have a simple reminder that can consistently point you in the direction of what you truly value. I have found that an easy way to do this is to imagine what you'd like others to say about you at your own funeral. What would you like to be known for? Write down a few phrases that come to mind. Do you want to be known for contributing something to the world, for being a great parent, for your career, for how you treated others? Whatever comes to mind is a good indication of what you especially value. I suggest you write down this information on a 3 x 5 card, and keep it near you. When deciding what to do with your time, you can refer to this card and ask yourself, "Would this (whatever you're thinking of doing) be a good use of my time considering who I want to be?"

- A second tool for prioritizing your life is to make a list of every goal you can think of. I call this your Master Goal List. It can be helpful to think of goals you have in various areas of your life, such as relationships, career, health, recreation, finances, spirituality, and hobbies. When you complete your master list of goals, you'll have a handy reference as to all the things you'd like to achieve. In daily life, some goals call loudly to us on a regular basis, such as financial matters, whereas spiritual or recreational goals are often relegated for the bottom of our "to do" list. By having your master list available, it'll be easier to be reminded of all the things you'd like to do. As you plan your days, you can look on your Master Goal List to see where you'd like to allocate your time.

- A third tool is to schedule yourself on a weekly or monthly basis, rather than just on a daily basis. When we schedule day-to-day, this helps us take care of what is necessary on a given day. Of course, many important things in life don't fit so well into a daily "to do" list. Vacations, special time with loved ones, activities or seminars that take more than just a day, and other events are best scheduled while looking at weekly or monthly calendars. I currently schedule time with friends, vacations, and spiritual retreats several months in advance. After all, I'm not completely booked up several months in advance, so it's easier for me to schedule things into my calendar when it's relatively empty. Then, when the time comes to be away, I've already blocked out the time. People who fail to schedule weeks or months in advance often find they only have time for urgent things, and that the nonurgent (but important) activities of life are crowded out.

- Another simple but great way to figure out the best use of your time is to ask yourself the question, "What's the bottleneck preventing me from having more fulfillment in my life?" A "bottleneck" is where energy is constricted—preventing things from moving forward at a more accelerated rate. It can be in virtually any area of life—career, finances, relationships, leisure time, spirituality, or personal goals. After asking yourself this question, see if you receive an intuitive answer that feels right. Once you know what your personal bottleneck to greater fulfillment is, you can focus on scheduling more time, energy, and possibly even more money on bettering this area of your life. Whatever you focus on tends to improve over time. Soon, your bottleneck may no longer be there, and a whole new level of fulfillment will be yours. Many years ago, I asked myself the "bottleneck question" and the answer was obvious. I needed more money. At the time, I was making about $5000 a year, and the lack of money in my life kept me from having the relationship I wanted, the ability to travel, and many other things. For several years, I focused on making more money—and it worked. Now, I have a new bottleneck. Since I'm in the habit of asking myself this question every few months, I avoided the pitfall of thinking that more money was *still* the bottleneck in my life. It's easy to not notice when the bottleneck in your life changes. By asking yourself this question periodically, you'll be able to change your priorities when it's called for, rather than many years after it's appropriate.

- Lastly, whenever you start a new project or commitment, in order to avoid becoming even busier in your life, *stop doing* some other activity you were doing before. Otherwise, your plate will be overfull. Once I realized the obvious logic of this concept, it was easier for me to say "no" to new opportunities that came my way, or to let go of old commitments. When a new situation came along that would require my time, I'd ask myself, "If I devote time to this new activity, what would I be willing to eliminate from my life in order to make room for it?" When evaluating that question, it often became clear that I wouldn't be willing to stop doing any of the things I was already doing. Therefore, I would decline the activity I was considering. Even when I ended up accepting the new commitment, I made sure I knew precisely what I would eliminate from my life.

Clarity is power. Knowing clearly what's important to you will help you make the best possible use of the time you have. Although the simple exercises offered here only take a few minutes, they can save you many hours spent on meaningless activities. When you spend your time doing activities fully in sync with your values, you'll feel less stress, less hurried, and better about your life.

5. Create Four Extra Hours a Day

Overcoming the Four Biggest Time Wasters

If time is money, four extra hours a day could be worth a lot of cash. Although almost everyone complains they don't have enough time, the truth is that, on average, people work no more today than they did twenty years ago. So where does all the time go? Much of it goes toward four major time wasters. Since life is more complicated than it was twenty years ago, these time wasters can eat away at your time much more than they used to. Unless you learn to get a handle on them, they can easily waste four or more hours each day.

1) The average American watches almost four and one-half hours of TV each and every day! Over the course of an average person's lifespan, they spend almost twelve years watching TV and only ten years at a job. Imagine how much more time you'd feel you had if you didn't watch any TV, or at least cut it down by half. If you're reading this book, you're probably not the type of person to watch four and a half hours a day. Yet, most people greatly underestimate how much TV they actually watch. You may think you only watch an hour a day, but when you consider sporting events, news, and weekend TV watching, the hours quickly add

up. Keeping a log of exactly how much TV you watch can be an eye-opening experience.

Once you have an idea of how much TV you watch, you may decide to change your habits. There are various ways to go about breaking the TV habit. You may try the cold turkey approach—simply unplug your TV. I did this about a year ago and I was amazed that in one simple action, my life was radically altered. I now had plenty of time to catch up on my reading, talk to friends, and pursue hobbies. If unplugging your TV sounds a bit radical, then you can choose, at the beginning of each week, the exact shows you plan to watch. It can be helpful to write down your selections on a note pad. Then, choose to watch only the shows you have previously selected, and nothing else. Simply by doing this one action, you'll likely gain at least an hour a day of extra time for more meaningful and rewarding activities.

2) The telephone. In modern life, the phone is obviously a necessity. Yet, the way most people use the telephone leads to an incredible waste of time. We answer the phone even when it's not convenient. We create idle chit-chat with people we don't even care about. We play prolonged "phone tag" because we fail to set telephone appointments. Fortunately, there are simple things you can do to save time on the phone, as well as simple ways to use the time you do spend on the phone more effectively.

In my opinion, the greatest time-saving technology you can buy is a 900 megahertz cordless phone with a headset attachment. You can get them at Radio Shack for under $100. A phone such as this allows the use of both of your hands while you walk around your house or office, and offers good, clear sound. You can clean your house, pay bills, do your laundry, or garden while talking to friends, family, and colleagues. This one device can easily save you an hour a day. Cellular phones can also help you save time by converting your time in the car or while waiting in line into productive time. While phones such as these can be a big time saver, be careful how you use them. Some calls, such as to those you love, are worth your full attention. As with any technology, you need to use such phones in a way that doesn't interfere with the quality of your life.

Besides having the right equipment, it's also important to use a phone wisely. Caller ID, available in many areas, can help you determine if you should pick up an incoming call, or simply let the machine get it. On an average day, I used to get seven calls from people trying to sell me something. Having Caller ID has helped me to avoid those calls. As with TV watching, keeping a phone log can be an eye-opening experience. For a week you can keep track of who you talked to and for how long. By looking over your log, you'll likely spot trends or people that are a waste of time. Another time-saving phone idea is to, at the beginning of a phone conversation, tell the person you're talking to, "I only have a couple of minutes to talk now. What can I help you with?" Saying a sentence such as that will encourage a brief, straight-to-the-point conversation. To politely curtail a conversation that is dragging on, you can say, "I have one last thing to say before I need to take off...." Such statements can help save a lot of time.

If you play phone tag as much as I used to, then you may want to start making telephone appointments. It's easy—just suggest two or three exact times someone can call you and likely find you available to talk when leaving a message on their machine or talking to their secretary. By leaving exact times, or requesting that they *tell you* a couple of times *they* would likely be available, you can save yourself endless rounds of messages. In order to be more efficient with your phone calls, it can help to bunch them all together. You can make your outgoing calls at the same time each day, and/or set aside an hour for taking calls. By doing this, the telephone won't be a distraction from your other work, and you can become more efficient in completing both your calls and your other work projects.

3) Disorganization. No one likes to take the time to organize their files, computer, office, desk, closet, and other aspects of modern-day life. However, disorganization is both a time waster and a constantly frustrating experience. Since it can seem overwhelming to organize all the different areas of your life, it's a good idea to focus on just one small area at a time. You might try spending an hour a week organizing a specific area of your life. Within a couple of months, you'll notice you can find things more easily, your head will seem clearer, and you'll be able to get more done in less time. What in your life would benefit by being more effectively organized? Make a commitment now to spend at least an hour in the upcoming week getting yourself better organized.

4) Waiting. We all lose a lot of time waiting—in traffic, in a bank line, at a doctor's office, or when put on hold on the phone. By planning ahead, you can turn such times into productive moments of your day. For example, if you have a cellular phone, you can return your calls. If you have reading material to catch up on, bring it with you to the bank or doctor's office. While driving, listen to audio books or self-help courses that can further your career or personal satisfaction. If you plan ahead, your "waiting" time can be well-spent time.

Obviously, there are more than just four time wasters we each contend with. Yet by reining in the four mentioned here, you'll be well on your way to creating "more" hours in your day. As you use your extra hours to further your financial and personal goals, you'll be rewarded with more prosperity, peace, and satisfying relationships.

6. Quickly Become an Expert

The Information Exchange Process

Until about a hundred years ago, most commerce was done by barter. People would exchange goods, services, or practical knowledge with each other, and in the process save a lot of time and money. Now, bartering is mostly a lost art. However, there are many advantages to it. I often get together with people who have expertise in an area I'm interested in, and exchange my expertise with theirs. This has often allowed me to acquire needed information or skills hundreds of times faster than I normally could learn. I call this method the "Information Exchange Process."

To make use of this process, I have written a one-page sheet that describes the reason, benefits, and structure of the Information Exchange. When I meet someone who has expertise in an area I would like to learn about, I give him or her this sheet. On the front side of the sheet is a description of the process. I have included here the description of this process I hand out to people. If you like the idea, you're welcome to copy my description. On the back of the paper I hand out, I list all the areas I feel I am an expert in. Usually, I simply hand this single sheet of paper to someone I'd like to learn from and say, "After reading this, give me a call if you're interested."

The Information Exchange Process

"I value learning a lot. Yet I've seen it often takes a long time to gain new skills and information. Therefore, I've come up with an extremely efficient way to become knowledgeable about new fields of interest: I call it an "Information Exchange" or I.E. for short. In the I.E. process, two people get together for the purpose of sharing their expertise with each other. For example, let's say you know a lot about buying a house, while I know a lot about hypnosis. If you were interested in learning more about hypnosis, and I wanted to learn how to buy a house, then we'd get together and exchange information and skills.

"There are several advantages to learning in this way. First of all, it's incredibly efficient. I have spent ten years studying hypnosis, but I could probably tell you everything I know about it in two hours, or give you a good understanding of it in five minutes. Now that's a true time saver! Other advantages of this type of exchange include the fact that they're fun, they deepen friendships, they reinforce our own knowledge, and they are a free and easy way to become a more expanded person.

"I decided to give you this idea and my enclosed list of skills because I respect you and your depth of knowledge. If the idea intrigues you, I invite you to read my list and circle the items you'd enjoy learning more about. Since I already know you in some manner, I already have a good idea of knowledge/skills you possess that I'd be interested in learning. The list I've enclosed consists of items in

which I can talk intelligently about for fifteen minutes or more. If you'd like to exchange information or skills with me, simply give me a call and tell me you're interested in doing an exchange. We could take it from there.

In having done this in the past, I've always been amazed by how well it works. The structure is this: after getting together, I'll talk and/or demonstrate a skill to you that you'd like to learn more about. After that's done, I'll make a specific request to learn something from you. So as to be fair, we each take about an equal time learning from the other person. In this way, the resources we've gathered can be shared for enhancing each other's lives. The whole process can usually be done over lunch, or even over the phone. I look forward to hearing from you. Call me at: (list your phone number).

Generally, people love the idea. Besides providing a simple way to learn new information at an accelerated rate, it's a great way to meet new people and form new friendships. Learning from someone who already knows the ins and outs of an area you'd like to learn about can literally save you years of struggle and time. During the exchange, you simply ask the other person to explain the essence of what they know about a particular topic or skill. You are encouraged to ask specific questions so you can find out the exact information you're looking for. Then, when you're done, they can ask about anything on your list.

Coming up with a list of items you're an expert on can be a bit challenging. Originally, I was able to come up with twenty such things. Yet as I asked my friends and family, "What do you consider me an expert on?" they suggested thirty-five other items. My list now contains fifty-five items, enough variety that almost anyone could find something they'd like to learn more about. Be sure to include things such as relationship skills, business skills, life lessons you've learned, hobbies, places you've traveled, etc.

Years ago, I needed to raise $45,000 for a video I wanted to do. I knew a friend who was good in business, and had previously secured a loan for starting his own company. In just thirty minutes he took me step-by-step through the whole process of writing a business plan, contacting investors, talking to banks, etc. During the next half-hour, I talked to him about how to meditate, improve his memory, and have more energy. That single hour transformed each of our lives. I raised the money, and the video ended up being very successful. He used the information I gave him to achieve greater health and peace. You can save countless time and energy learning from "experts" using the Information Exchange process. Try it, you'll like it.

7. Work Fewer Hours

Cold Turkey Time Management

Joe Brinkley's wife had been complaining about his long hours at work for years. But now Joe and Betty were in my office for divorce counseling. Betty laid out her position by stating, "If Joe decides to work more than forty hours a week ever again, I'm going to file for an immediate divorce." I could tell Betty was serious, and so could Joe. Joe adored Betty, but then again, he also adored his job. His reasons and excuses for working up to sixty-five hours a week fell on deaf ears. I told him that if he wanted to save his marriage, he was going to have to free himself from working so much. Thus, the "Cold Turkey" approach to working fewer hours was born.

Joe agreed to be home by 6:00 P.M. every day, or else face Betty's determined exit. In a private counseling session with me, he asked for advice on how to change his ways. I had two suggestions. First, I suggested he get a watch that had a multiple alarm function, and set it for 5:00 P.M. That would remind him that he had thirty minutes before he had to begin his drive home. Then, I advised him to set the second alarm for 5:30. No matter what he was doing when he heard that alarm, even if he was in the middle of a meeting, I advised him to pick up his briefcase, and drive home. That's it. A simple decision, a simple commitment, and no room for excuses.

The second suggestion I made to Joe was to have one hour a day assigned as his "priority hour." During this hour, he would do whatever he considered as his long-term priority tasks, with absolutely no interruptions. No telephone calls, no people barging in, no snacks, no nothing. I advised Joe to tell everyone in his office when this hour would be each day, and get them trained to respect it. That way, Joe could make sure the most important tasks got done each day, and that he could handle them when he was focused.

Joe took my advice, and it immediately threw his work situation into chaos. During the first week, he found himself having to leave in the middle of important meetings, phone calls, and presentations. He had to remind people not to interrupt him when the "Do Not Disturb" sign was on his door. Yet Betty was happy, and he wanted to keep her happy. The lack of flexibility of his commitment forced Joe to change how he did things at the office. He finally began to delegate, something he was never good at before. He began to spend less time on trivial items, and instead focused on the most important things that only he could do. He even started to pace his day so that when 5:00 P.M. rolled around, there were just a couple of minor things to do before driving home. Both Betty and I were impressed!

Meanwhile, in my own life, I wanted to work fewer hours too. Although I didn't have someone like Betty pushing me toward a do-or-die situation, I decided I only wanted to work thirty-five hours a week (down from forty-five). Like Joe, my first week was crazy. I often wondered, "Why am I turning off my computer right before the article is complete?" Still, I kept to my commitment—even when it made no sense. By the second week, my mind had subconsciously figured out what I needed to do to work ten fewer hours a week. I even set up a priority hour, and found that once I could successfully ignore a ringing phone, I could accomplish an enormous amount in an hour.

You probably know a lot about prioritizing your day. You've likely read various time-management ideas. The advantage of the Cold Turkey method is that, when all else fails to rein in your time, this technique works. It forces you to change how you structure your day and handle your time by creating a bottom-line change. It's amazingly effective, and can be used in association with various other techniques. The hardest thing about using this method is the fact that you probably don't have Betty threatening you! Therefore, you're going to need to create your own threat. Fortunately, vee have vays of making you do vat you say you vant to do! If you really want to work fewer hours, I suggest you rip up $10 for each hour you work more than your stated commitment.

Most people who work fifty or more hours a week do so, not because they need the money, but because they are addicted to work. Sure, there are always plenty of reasons for working more. For many people, the bottom line is that they have a hard time leaving the office and focusing on the other parts of their life. One way to help an addict become free is by making their old behavior immediately painful. The act of tearing up $10 for each extra hour one works has the effect of persuading people to keep to their commitments. I've used this with many clients, and in each case it has soon worked. For about $40 of ripped-up money, even workaholic executives have managed to work far fewer hours. Now that's a pretty good deal.

If you'd like to work fewer hours, consider making your own commitment to these methods. Simply set up the amount of time you'd like to work each day, and the penalty for each extra hour you work. From experience, I suggest ripping up money as a good penalty because it has proven so effective in getting people to change their behavior. If $10 an hour is too much, decide on an amount you'd be willing to rip up if you break your promise. In addition, decide if you might want to set up your own priority hour, and begin this commitment by telling all the people in your office. The effect these tools can have on your life are immense. Not only will you have more time to take care of yourself, but the people you care about will also be rewarded. Are you ready to commit?

8. Keep Your Life on Track

The Six Questions of Success

If someone asked me to describe in four simple words how they could achieve wealth, health, and happiness, my answer would be easy: ask the right questions. When we ask ourselves good questions, it leads us to make better decisions as to where and how to spend our time. When we fail to ask the right questions, we can easily fall prey to mechanical routines, other people's goals, and a life of unhappiness. When it comes to taking charge of your time and your life, asking the right questions can be the answer you've been looking for.

I have previously written two books that consist primarily of questions. After *The Little Book of Big Questions* became the focus of an Oprah Winfrey show, I received many letters from people telling me how the inquiries in the book had helped shape their life. People would tell me which were their favorite questions, and why. From that and other feedback, I created a list of six questions that seemed the most valuable in gently guiding people back to the life they truly desired. I have found that answering these questions once a month can be an amazingly efficient way to create the life you really want. Traditionally, around New Year's people often look back on their life to see what's working and what isn't. Asking the following list of six questions is similar, except these are designed to precisely guide you in a way to gain maximum benefit. In addition, because so much is always going on nowadays, it's helpful to evaluate things on a monthly (rather than yearly) basis.

When answering these questions, it's best to say your answers out loud to a mate, friend, or coworker. Another option is to write down what you have to say in a journal. Somehow, saying the answers out loud or writing things down has more impact than simply thinking them in your head. You may find that some questions require a fair amount of thought or reflection to properly answer, while others will seem simple or obvious.

For each of the six questions that follow, I give a brief description of why it can be useful to ask yourself, or those you love, this question once a month. Then, I provide my own brief answer to each of these inquiries (in italics) so you can better understand how they can be useful for guiding a person's life:

1) What can I do this week to bring more fun and/or meaning into my life?

As adults, most of us get lost in daily routines, problems, and plans. Yet when we were children, life was very different. We're not born into this world as planners and problem solvers, but as bundles of playful energy. This question can help remind you to schedule something each week to bring fun and/or meaning into your life. It will help provoke your thinking as to what you currently find fun or meaningful, and help you keep these things as priorities in your life. My answer:

I'd like to go mountain biking with Michelle this week. I'm going to put it down in my schedule to call her. If she can't go biking, then perhaps I could get some friends together to play Pictionary. Also, I'd like to begin reading the book Tuesdays with Morrie. *A couple of friends have told me it's very thought-provoking and touching, and I think that would be an easy way to be inspired during the week.*

2) What could I feel grateful for in my life?

This may seem like a strange question to get your life in order, but it's important to remember what is going great in your life. If you focus only on what's wrong with your life, you'll always be thinking about problems. Part of living a successful life means focusing on what's going well, and feeling grateful for how blessed you are. Unfortunately, it's all too easy to forget to count your blessings. This question will help you to remember to do just that. When answering this question, try to come up with more than just intellectual answers. Instead, attempt to really *feel* grateful for what you have in your life. Feeling grateful for the people, events, work, luxuries, and other things in your life is a shortcut to feeling wealthy, healthy, and happy. My answer:

I am so thankful that my back doesn't hurt anymore. My body feels good. I am grateful that my dog is no longer sick, and that we've been having a great time together. I feel really lucky to be living where I am, and have so many caring friends around me. I am also grateful to be able to do a job I truly enjoy.

3) How can I use the gifts I've been given to better serve people?

If you want to make a lot of money, get good at giving people what they want. If you want love, become skillful at caring for people. If you want to grow spiritually, get good at helping people. Whatever you want in life, you can receive it by becoming good at serving people. This question will help you to consistently ponder how you can do this more effectively. Even small actions done consistently can make a world of difference.

As a counselor, I often see how it's the little things that make or break a relationship. I often give couples this question as a way to make sure they consistently treat people well. I have found that the people who make helping and caring for others a priority are the ones who become most successful in life. My answer:

I could tell my friends and family about positive changes I've seen in them, as well as specific things I admire about them. I could use my gift for lightness and humor to inspire people to enjoy life. I could send my former clients a newsletter with helpful tips on how to set goals for the new year.

4) Is there anything I'm doing that is hurting myself, other people, or steering me off course?

When planes fly to a destination, they are off course over 90 percent of the time. However, they almost constantly correct their course so they end up where they're supposed to be. We need to do likewise. When people make mistakes, they often spend a lot of time in blame, self-pity, or distraction. That just makes matters worse. Instead, what we need to do is quickly realize when we're off course, and immediately take the actions necessary to get back on track. My answer:

I haven't been exercising enough, and I've been eating more sweets than I would like. I think I need to leave more time in my schedule to be by myself in nature. In fact, I'm going to make sure I do that this week.

5) On a scale of 1 to 10, with 10 being the best possible, how are the following areas of my life currently going?

a) Finances   d) Level of fulfillment   f) Spirituality

b) Career   e) Body/health   h) Personal goals

c) Relationships

Whatever you can measure, you can improve. Since measuring one's financial status is rather easy, people often get overly focused on this area of life. Yet, by simply rating all the areas above on a 1 to 10 scale, you can get a quick assessment of how each aspect of your life is going. I've seen that a person's quality of life is often determined by how the worst thing in their life is going. For example, if a person is rich, but of poor health, their quality of life will be determined much more by their health than by their wealth. By evaluating on a monthly basis how each aspect of your life is proceeding, you'll be better able to make adjustments in how you spend your time and energy.

6) What would be good to do to create more balance, harmony, or growth in my life?

Your answer to this question should naturally proceed from how you evaluated the various aspects of your life in the previous inquiry. If you realized that most aspects of your life were working well—except your relationships—then you could focus on how to improve your relationships. To answer this question, it helps to access your intuition, or the still, small voice inside. Perhaps there has been something you've been avoiding, and this question will help you realize it's time to move forward. Whenever possible, try to be specific with your answer and the new action(s) you plan to take. Insights are helpful, but only changes in actual behavior are likely to lead to the results you desire. My answer:

I'd like to focus more attention on feeling spiritually at peace. One way I could do that would be to go to the redwoods and camp out a couple of days. Also, I'd like to spend more time listening to my favorite spiritual music and doing yoga. I think I could grow personally by being more vulnerable with my friends about my feelings.

These six questions are an easy, quick, and powerful way to gain important insights that will help you plan your time wisely. Rather than waiting until a problem is big, these questions will help you to handle things when they're small and easily handled. By writing your answers in a journal, or taking turns answering these questions with a friend, you can help each other create the life you truly desire.

WHY IS IT THAT I'M MOST AWARE OF MY BODY ONLY WHEN IT'S NOT WORKING PROPERLY?

Ashleigh Brilliant

Secrets to Health

It's hard to feel good about life when you're not feeling healthy. When we have our health, we tend to take it for granted, but when we have a cold, flu, or something worse, it becomes our whole life. Rather than wait for a disease or chronic ailment to spur us into action, it's a good idea to try to maintain good health by engaging in simple, preventative measures. The adage "an ounce of prevention is worth a pound of cure" couldn't be more true than in the area of health care. Even corporations are learning they can save money by providing their employees with preventive health care. A few minutes a day of effective health strategies can help you avoid weeks of illness, medical costs, and even an early death.

Since the dominant medical model in the Western world has been the treatment of sickness rather than the maintenance of health, many of the ideas in this section are relatively unknown. However, in other parts of the world, such as China, if a patient gets sick, they fire their doctor—after all, they see it as the doctor's job to make sure they *don't* get sick! Therefore, doctors in such countries have developed a variety of methods to make sure people stay healthy. As you practice some of these strategies, you'll find that you'll feel healthier, stronger, and less susceptible to things like winter colds or flus. In addition, as you gain vitality and avoid sickness, you'll be able to use your extra time and energy to find success in the other areas of your life.

9: Get Healthy and Energized

The Science of Supplements

As recently as a hundred years ago, most people in the world grew their own food. Now, only 1 percent of Americans are farmers. As we've entered an era of fertilizers, pesticides, and genetically engineered crops, the quality and quantity of nutrients in our foods has gone down. Fortunately, at the same time, we've developed vitamin and mineral supplements that can help us get the nutrition we need. Almost weekly, scientists are announcing that another vitamin or supplement has been found to reduce the chance of heart disease, Alzheimer's, cancer, or some other affliction. Yet faced with more information than we can stand, many of us simply tune out and avoid the whole subject. Unfortunately, in the area of health and nutrition, ignorance is not bliss. In fact, ignorance can lead to chronic disease or an early death. I am not a doctor and cannot make specific recommendations for you, but here's what I have found to be personally helpful.

I always take a vitamin and mineral supplement. I like Twinlabs Daily One Cap without iron. For less than 30 cents a day, this single pill provides many of the basic vitamins and minerals you need. If you're willing to spend more money and take three pills a day, I like Rainbow Lite's Master Nutrient System. This is an excellent vitamin and mineral supplement which is "food based." Basically, this means that it is derived from foods, and can therefore be better utilized by your body than synthetic vitamins. Both of these products are available in most health food stores.

The good thing about vitamin pills is their convenience. It only takes a few seconds a day to provide your body with its needed nutrients. Yet, I prefer to drink my vitamins in a glass of juice or in a smoothie because the powdered form usually provides higher doses of nutrients. In addition, I've noticed that I often immediately feel energized after drinking a powder-based vitamin formula. My favorite powder-based vitamin and mineral formula is called All-One. It comes in various formulas, but the one I enjoy is called Green Phyto Based All-One. I start each morning with a tablespoon in a cup of juice, blended with half a banana. It tastes great, gives me more energy than a cup of coffee, and my body sings with delight. Not bad for under $1 a day.

Another great powder formula is called The Ultimate Meal. This product provides you with all the vitamins, minerals, and antioxidants you could possibly want. If you don't have time to eat, or if you want large doses of everything your body might need, The Ultimate Meal would be a good way to go. It costs about $2 per serving. Once again, you can find these powder formulas in most health food stores, but if you have a hard time finding them, you can call All-One at (800) 235-5727 or The Ultimate Meal at (800) 843-6325. Their respective web sites are: www.All-one.com and www.ultimatelife.com.

I also take an antioxidant supplement. Antioxidant formulas include various ingredients that have been shown to reduce the likelihood of cancer, heart disease, and arthritis, as well as slow the aging process. A company called Country Life has a great product called Super 10 Antioxidant. For about 80 cents a day, the ingredients in this formula may help prevent some of the worse health problems Westerners typically face, such as heart disease and cancer. Although most health food stores carry Country Life, you can also call (800) 645-5768.

If you want to feel even more vitality, consider replacing the coffee you drink with a product called Uptime. As I mentioned in my previous book *Shortcuts to Bliss,* Uptime has a very small amount of caffeine in it, but mostly consists of various things that are good for you, such as vitamin C, blue-green algae, and wheat grass. Just like a cup of coffee, Uptime can make you feel energized but without the jittery feeling or crash that can happen when you drink coffee. The people at Uptime even have an "energy bar" called Peanut Butter and Jelly that's like a candy bar, but it's healthy for you and gives you energy. You can order Uptime products by calling (800) 441-5656 or reach them on the Web at: www.up-time.com. Many people also report that locally grown bee pollen makes them feel better and energized. In addition, there are now many juice bars around the country that offer smoothies filled with energy enhancing products. Sipping on one throughout the day is likely to help you to feel dynamic, healthy, and fully alive.

Lastly, to prevent heart disease (the number one killer in America), consider asking your doctor if he or she recommends you take an aspirin each day. Many studies have shown that very low dosages of aspirin can prevent a first heart attack, or can help keep you alive in case of a heart attack. Since your risk of heart disease and tolerance to aspirin are best decided by your doctor, it's a good idea to seek professional guidance on this matter.

In the area of health, the little things you consistently do can make a big difference later on in your life. Consult with your preferred medical personnel and decide on what you'd be willing to commit to do each day. Once you find the right supplements to fit into your time, budgetary, and commitment requirements, stay with the program.

10: Overcome Insomnia

You are Getting Sleepy…

Insomnia is a hidden epidemic in our culture. It affects one in three people on a fairly regular basis. In Western society, the traditional remedy is to take sleeping pills. However, all prescription sleeping pills interfere with normal sleep patterns, and can even be physically addictive. The answer to insomnia is not to be found in pills, but rather in some common-sense remedies and some simple internal methods to help you fall asleep.

Most insomnia is caused by a buildup of stress during the day. If you live a stressful life, and fail to take periodic "relaxation breaks" during the day, you are more prone to being wide awake when it's time to go to bed. Simple relaxation techniques such as deep breathing, a leisurely walk, or listening to a calming tape or CD during the day can help alleviate a buildup of anxiety. These same things can also be useful right before you go to bed.

However, if you have a history of insomnia, or if you are experiencing a particularly stressful time in your life, you may need something more. Fortunately, there are ways to lull yourself to sleep that don't involve pills.

As a licensed hypnotist, I see a lot of people in my private practice who complain of insomnia. I have found that 90 percent of these people can be helped by using one of two simple methods. The first technique I call The Blackboard Countdown, and the second I call The Hypnotic Bore. In The Blackboard Countdown (TBC), after crawling into bed, picture a blackboard in your mind with the number 1000 on it. Imagine erasing the number, and then seeing the words *Deep Asleep* written on it. Imagine erasing the words *Deep Asleep,* and then picture the number 999 on the board. Erase the number and picture *Deep Asleep* once again. Keep counting back, followed by *Deep Asleep*. If you ever lose track as to what number you're on, simply start over at 1000.

The Blackboard Countdown is a bit like counting sheep, but it's much more potent. The reason it's effective is due to the hypnotic rhythm it creates, an endless repetition of going from counting, back to the suggestion *Deep Asleep,* over and over again. It requires just enough concentration to keep your mind occupied, but not enough to actually keep you entertained. Studies show that after only five minutes of this type of meditative mental activity, your heart rate, blood pressure, and breathing rate equals that of normal sleep. What this means is that even if you don't fall asleep right away, your body will be receiving as much rest as if you were actually asleep. Since this method requires no pills or gadgets to carry, you can use it anywhere, anytime. Many people are surprised by the results.

If The Blackboard Countdown doesn't work for you after a couple of tries, I suggest trying what I call The Hypnotic Bore method. I used to have a math teacher who could put anyone to sleep. Even after drinking a couple of cups of coffee, I'd be off in la-la land after just a few minutes of hearing him pontificate. He seemed to have the same effect on everyone else in the class. I surmised that it was something about his voice. He spoke in a slow monotone that never had any rhythm, emphasis, or speed. Unfortunately, I never recorded his voice, so I can't sell you tapes of his talking to help with occasional insomnia. It's too bad, because it surely would have worked. However, the next best thing is to record your own voice into a cassette recorder, and play it back to yourself when you have the need. Below is a transcript of what to say into the recorder. It's important that you speak very, very, very slowly, and with a constant monotone:

"Take a deep breath and let out any tension with your breath. Take another deep breath, and once again relax fully as you exhale. Notice any part of your body that feels a bit tight or uncomfortable, and see if you can relax that part of your body as you exhale. Check your legs and make sure they feel comfortable and relaxed. Notice your arms, and see if they feel comfortable and relaxed. Imagine breathing a favorite soothing color deep into your lungs, and feel how it relaxes and soothes you with each breath you take. Allow the feeling of relaxation to soothe your jaw, cheek, and forehead muscles. Good. Now imagine that you're at the top of a flight of stairs, and as I count back from 100, with each number I count back, you'll feel more relaxed and tired. Eventually you will simply drift off into a peaceful, restful sleep."

(As you begin the countdown, following the form given below, have your voice grow increasingly soft and slow, until by the time you're at 30, it should be a slow whisper.)

"100. Imagine yourself slowly walking down some stairs to a deeper level of rest and relaxation. 99. With each number I count back you feel like you are drifting into a restful sleep. 98. You can put aside any thoughts or concerns, knowing that you can easily handle things in the morning. 97. All your thoughts are drifting farther away, as if on a cloud, leaving you more and more tired. 96. Deeper and deeper with each number. 95. Letting go even more. 94. Your whole body and mind feeling so tired. 93. You are already experiencing a deeper rest and relaxation. 92. You will soon simply drift off into a restful sleep. 91. Drifting off into a deep, sound sleep."

The above countdown should take several minutes. When continuing the countdown all the way to zero, just use the above transcript, but substitute the number 90 (then 80, 70, etc.) for the number 100. For example, the next part of the countdown would be: "90. Imagine yourself slowly walking down some stairs to a deeper level of rest and relaxation. 89...." Remember to speak softer (or hold the tape recorder a bit farther away) with each group of ten that you count back. That will make it easier for you to simply drift off into a natural sleep.

When you have the tape recorded, buy what's called a pillow speaker (about $5 at Radio Shack). This is a small, flat speaker that fits under your pillow. When you are having a hard time getting to sleep, simply put the tape in a Walkman, put the pillow speaker under your pillow, and let your own monotonous voice lull you to sleep. Many people report that using a Hypnotic Bore tape results in a particularly good night's sleep. And once you have established your regular sleeping pattern, you'll feel better about yourself and have more time to enjoy life. Sweet dreams.

11: Revitalize Your Body in Three Minutes

The Three-Minute Body Miracle

It's a rainy, sleepy afternoon, and you're stuck in front of your computer. Your bones are weary, your eyes blurry, and your mind feels burned out. You can grab another cup of coffee, but you know your body really doesn't need any more caffeine. What to do? If you knew that in three minutes of effort you could go from burned out to blissed out, would it be worth your while? If the answer is yes, then the Three-Minute Body Miracle (or T.M.B.M for short) is for you. This simple, but amazingly effective four-step technique does several things in a short period of time. First, it gets your body naturally energized. Second, it stimulates blood flow to the brain for better focus and concentration. And finally, it allows you to quickly let go of stress and tension in both your body and mind. If you try it just a couple of times, I think you'll be hooked.

Since most people work at jobs in which they sit for large periods of time (as I do), step one is to stand up and shake your body. Our bodies were not meant to sit for long periods of time. It makes our joints hurt and our muscles tighten. By shaking your shoulders, arms, legs, and hips for a mere one minute, you can stimulate energy and blood flow throughout your body. During your minute of shaking, make sure you vigorously move both your arms, shoulders, and legs. Pretend you're a rag doll, and you're able to shake the tension right out.

You may feel embarrassed shaking your body vigorously for a full minute. If you are afraid of other people seeing you, close your office door, or go to the bathroom. Children move and shake all the time because it's a natural desire of our bodies to do so. Yet as adults we've become accustomed to being sedentary. Unfortunately, not moving leads to feeling even more tired, which leads to even less movement. Breaking out of this cycle is easier than you think. The main obstacles are laziness and fear of embarrassment. Since this entire process takes only three minutes (and only one minute of shaking), there's no good excuse for not doing it. Once you try this method a couple of times, you'll get over your initial embarrassment because you'll be too busy feeling good.

The second step is to imagine you're on a trampoline, and bounce up and down on your toes for thirty seconds. By doing this, you help to counteract the force of gravity that can make you feel tired and help stimulate your lymph glands and immune system. It's like giving your body an internal massage. The third step is to energetically massage your ears, face, and scalp for another thirty seconds or so. Your ears, face, and scalp are loaded with acupressure points that help to relax, energize, and balance your entire body. With practice you'll learn what feels best, but the basic idea is to vigorously and quickly rub every square inch of your head. When briefly massaging your ears, you can knead your ears between your thumbs and other fingers. When rubbing your face and scalp, you can use the tips of all eight of your fingers and move them in rapid, small circular motions all over your head. This motion will help to release all the tension you hold in your face and scalp, as well as stimulate a nice, tingling, and warm feeling throughout your head.

Once you're done massaging your head, you should take a very deep breath, tighten your shoulders by bringing them to your ears, and hold your breath for ten seconds. When you let go of your breath, exhale with a loud sighing sound as you feel the release of your shoulders. Focus for a moment on the feeling of warmth in your shoulders and face. Finally, think of something or someone you feel grateful for. It could be your pet, your child, your health, your house, virtually anything. Feel a sense of gratitude in your heart for having this person, animal, or thing in your life. For a few moments, imagine you can breathe through your heart and have your gratitude expand with each and every breath. When you're ready, slowly open your eyes and notice how relaxed and energized you feel.

Many people do the Three Minute Body Miracle as a substitute for a coffee break, a bite to eat, or a cigarette. By substituting this method for something unhealthy, such as a candy bar, you can help yourself lose weight and become energized at the same time. Another advantage of this method is that it helps to make you more focused and alert. I've noticed that by doing this when I first feel tired in the afternoon, I can continue to be productive, rather than half-asleep. I literally gain an extra hour each day of alert, productive time by practicing this technique twice a day. Once again, the T.M.B.M. consists of four simple steps:

1. Stand up and shake every part of your body for a minute.

2. Bounce up and down on your toes for thirty seconds.

3. Vigorously massage your ears, face, and head for about thirty more seconds.

4. Take a deep breath, tighten your shoulders for ten seconds while holding your breath, exhale with a loud sigh and let your shoulders relax. Focus on some person, animal or thing you could feel grateful for. Feel the gratitude in your heart.

As a reminder to do this method, put a Post It note by your computer or on your desk. You can also get in the habit of doing it during your lunch break, or first thing upon coming home from work. Feel free to explore your own unique ways to fully enjoy the body shake-out, the massage, and the gratitude sections of this exercise. This method can even be used to get you out of stuck feelings or unhealthy thoughts that are bothering you. Its uses are almost endless, but unless you try it a couple of times, you'll never know how effective it can be. Therefore, I recommend you try it now, while the method is still fresh in your head. Don't do it halfway. Instead, do it with exaggerated passion and energy. You'll be surprised at how much better you can feel in three minutes. And your body will thank you.

12: Keep In Great Shape

The Skill of Exercise Selection

There is a proven exercise that is more effective in keeping you in great shape than all other forms of exercise. It is so much better than the alternatives, there isn't even a close second. The type of exercise proven to be the most effective is the one that you'll *actually do.* No matter what gym you belong to or what exercise skills you know about, they are all useless unless you consistently use them. That's why I think it's much better to do a mediocre exercise program that is fun, rather than a difficult, complex program that you rarely practice. In the game of getting and staying in shape, consistency wins.

There's a well-known psychological principle that says, "people do things to avoid pain and/or gain pleasure." Unfortunately, for most people, exercise is painful—therefore they avoid it. It's next to impossible to get yourself to consistently do exercise that you hate. What's needed is an exercise plan that is doable. Many people, once they feel out of shape, resolve to begin an exercise program that is unrealistic. They set a goal of doing four hours of hard exercise a week, when they haven't done four hours of exercise in the last six months! Such a plan is bound to fail. Instead, I suggest that people start slowly and easily. If during the last week you didn't do any exercise, try doing ten minutes this upcoming week. It will feel good if you can truly complete your stated goal. Then, build on your success. Next week, do twenty minutes of exercise, then thirty, and so on. Within two months, you can be up to thirty minutes of exercise three times a week, which is what many experts suggest is the minimum of what we need.

What to do? Basically, there are three types of exercise: body building (such as lifting weights), aerobic (such as running), and stretching (such as hatha yoga). An ideal program includes some of each of these three different forms of exercise. Yet, anything is better than nothing, so do whatever you find minimally painful, or even fun to do. It's also helpful to create a routine that works well for you. I used to jog as my primary form of exercise. I hated it, so I rarely did it. Then, I asked myself a key question: "What could I do to make my exercise more fun or less difficult?" As I thought about it, I came up with various answers:

1. I could listen to music or audio books while I exercise.

2. I could ride my bike to a nice nature spot, instead of run on the street.

3. I could take a brisk walk with a friend.

4. I could have a cup of coffee before I exercise.

5. When I use a stationary cycle, I could read a favorite magazine, or watch TV.

6. I could immediately reward myself with a type of food I like after I exercise.

7. I could exercise along with fun exercise videos.

You may be able to take advantage of some of the ideas on my list, or make up your own suggestions for making exercise more enjoyable. For some people, paying money to a gym is helpful in getting them to be consistent. In addition, many gyms have aerobic type classes that are fun. If there is a form of exercise that you're blessed to enjoy, such as biking, swimming, or roller blades, invest in the proper equipment. I've noticed that when a person buys a bike or an exercise machine, they feel obligated to use it.

I have repeatedly mentioned in this book that the key to success is balance. As it is with your life, so it is with your body. Surprisingly, studies show that a lot of exercise isn't much better for your body than just thirty minutes, three times a week. Similarly, sprinting isn't any better than jogging, nor is lifting a lot of weight better than lifting moderate amounts. Go easy on yourself and your body. That will make it easier on you, and easier to maintain the consistency you desire. In order to do your body the most good, try to spend some time each week practicing stretching, body building, and aerobic training (where you increase your heart rate). Many people find that a routine of five minutes of stretching, followed by twenty minutes of aerobic activity, followed by five more minutes of stretching is a good thirty-minute workout. Then, on other days of exercise, they focus on stretching combined with body building.

If you've put off practicing a consistent exercise program in the past, decide what you'd be willing to start doing this week. Build on your successes each week, and try new things till you find what works best for you. Schedule it into your week. Your appointment to do your exercise is just as important as an appointment you make with your doctor or dentist. If you use the principles outlined here, you'll soon be amazed at how easy it is to consistently exercise. In just a few short weeks your body will look and feel a whole lot better.

13: Avoid A Cold or Flu

The Wonders of Immune Supplements

I used to have a girlfriend who was an acupuncturist. She introduced me to the Eastern approach to medicine, which is decidedly different than in the West. Rather than thinking in terms of which approach is better, I looked to see how I might prevent getting a cold or flu using the best each had to offer. I used to frequently get a cold or flu, and I was sick and tired of being sick and tired. Using the following ideas, I've only been sick for six days over the past three years. Although some of the suggestions I'll be making involve paying for supplements, their cost is low, especially considering the alternative. If you work for yourself (as I do), and make a decent income, each day of being sick can cost you much more than a hundred dollars. Usually, that's enough to buy a year's supply of immune-boosting supplements to make sure you stay healthy.

To begin with, in order to stay healthy you don't need to avoid being around people who are sick. Cold and flu viruses are always around us and in us. It is only when our immune system is weakened that we can't fight off their effects on our body. One way we weaken our immune system is by eating foods high in sugar or partially hydrogenated oils (found in much junk food). It's no coincidence that people often get sick around the holiday season at the same time they are devouring apple pies and Christmas cookies. If you tend to get sick at certain times of the year, try eating less junk food and more fruits and vegetables at those times.

Of course, when an apple pie is in front of me, I tend to forget all this. Therefore, I have a backup plan for myself. By taking supplements to keep my immune system strong, I make it more difficult for typical viruses to take hold in my body. Vitamin C has been proven to help prevent colds, as well as make their effects less severe. Between 1,000 and 2,000 milligrams a day seems to work for me. If possible, get vitamin C with bioflavanoids from several sources in it. For even better immune-boosting ability, there is a supplement called Advanced Defense System Plus by the Rainbow Lite company. It costs about $1 a day. If you're especially prone to sickness during a certain month or season, such as winter, consider taking these tablets as a simple way to build up your immune system. Rainbow Lite products are available in many health food stores, or by calling (800) 635-1233.

A second step to avoid getting sick is to take good care of yourself. Researchers estimate that over 80 percent of illnesses are due to stress. You probably already have things you do to combat stress, but the important thing is to be consistent in doing them. The basics of a healthy body are eating right, getting plenty of sleep, exercise, and relaxation. Even when I'm incredibly busy, I make sure not to let these things slide. After all, I'd just end up sick, and then be even more behind than I was before. Therefore, I keep to a certain standard of sleep, exercise, and relaxation, and make sure they are not crowded out by my busy schedule.

If you feel the first signs of a cold or flu coming on, there are several things you can do to lessen or eliminate the symptoms in a healthy way. Instead of taking an antihistamine or other cold remedy that simply *masks* the symptoms, the following supplements can actually help your body stay healthy. The one which has received a lot of attention lately is zinc lozenges. Several studies have shown that zinc gluconate can, when taken at the first symptoms of a cold, greatly reduce the severity of symptoms. I recommend Twinlabs zinc lozenges, but almost any one with zinc gluconate will do.

Many Eastern cultures think of colds differently than we do here. In the West, doctors say we get colds due to contracting a virus, while in the East they see it as an imbalance of *chi* or life-force energy. To help a person get back into balance, they often use something called *Yin Chiao*. I love this stuff. Whenever I have the very first symptoms of a cold, I take a few of these pills and I usually sidestep actually getting a cold. My friends and I have often been amazed at how well this supplement works. Although some health food stores carry it, most don't. The best way to get it is to mail order it from Vitamins 4 Less. Their toll-free number is (888) 782-8482. Ask for the *Yin Chiao* (pronounced "chow") with echinacea by Planetary Formula. It costs about $8, plus shipping charges.

Last, but not least, I want to mention how you can avoid getting the flu. Nothing is more debilitating than a flu virus that knocks you out. Fortunately, there is a lot that can be done to avoid such unpleasantness. To begin with, there are now flu vaccines that work pretty well. Since your risk of getting a flu versus the price and risk of taking the vaccine is best determined by your doctor, it's best to contact him or her for a professional opinion. In addition, a lot of people report very positive results with a homeopathic remedy by a company called Boiron. The exact name of the product you want to get is Oscillococcinum. I don't name these things, I only report on them. Anyway, when I have felt the first symptoms of a flu, such as fever, chills, or body aches, I've taken these pills and headed the virus off at the pass. It really seems to work. You can get this stuff at many health food stores, or at the Vitamins 4 Less number given above. It costs about $12.

When we have our health, we tend to take it for granted. Yet when we're sick, we realize there is nothing more important than good health. Knowing and *using* the information provided here to prevent colds and flus will add quality to your life.

14: Easily Stop Smoking

Secrets to a Smoke-Free Life

If you smoke, you know you should quit. After all, smoking kills more people than all other addictive drugs combined. So why do you smoke? Simply put, nicotine is the most addictive drug in the world. You fear going through withdrawals, losing a "friend" who has always been there for you, and feeling nervous. But quitting smoking is worth it. The average smoker dies ten years earlier than nonsmokers. Nowadays, if you smoke, you're constantly inconvenienced since you're not allowed to smoke in many places. Then there's the issues of how you smell, secondhand smoke, and on and on. Fortunately, quitting smoking doesn't have to be that hard, especially if you follow the step-by-step guidelines I offer. Ten years ago I created a video, *60 Minutes to a Smoke Free Life*. I still receive grateful letters from people who are surprised that they were able to quit.

The first step to ending this bad habit is to increase your motivation for quitting by writing what I call a "pain/pleasure essay." Write down the emotional and physical pain smoking has caused you in the past, and is causing you now. Be specific and graphic. For example, write about the times people gave you weird looks and you were embarrassed, or about the times you found yourself out of breath while walking up a couple of flights of stairs. If your family or friends want you to quit, include how uncomfortable their pleas make you feel. Then, write about all the potential pain continuing to smoke may cause you in the future. Life expectancy as a smoker is age sixty-two for men, and for women, sixty-five. Perhaps you can think about how painful it would be to have your young grandchildren at your hospital bed, crying as they watch you die, and you realizing you could have prolonged your life. As I said, be specific and graphic.

Next, write about all the pleasure you'll receive as a result of taking charge of your body and health. Even after one year of not smoking, your chances of a heart attack are cut in half! Perhaps friends and family will congratulate you, you'll have more energy, and you'll feel great about what you've accomplished. Write down whatever comes to mind. Then, once a day until a week after you quit, read your pain/pleasure essay. It will only take a couple of minutes to read, but it will help keep you motivated when you most need it.

The next step to quitting cigarettes is to discover smoking substitutes. Below a list of seven simple things you can do instead of smoke:

1. Eat carrot or celery sticks.

2. Take a warm shower or bath.

3. Watch TV or rent a video.

4. Go for a brisk walk or exercise.

5. Chew gum or enjoy a Life Savers candy (you can suck air through the hole).

6. Call a friend.

7. Listen to music and/or get up and dance.

Another great thing to do instead of smoke is something I call the Relaxation Breath. In just forty seconds, this unique method can take you from stressed out to fully relaxed. It can come in handy when you really want a cigarette. The technique is simple: when you feel a desire for a cigarette, take as deep a breath as you can, and hold it for ten seconds. When you exhale, let out a slow, sighing sound. Then picture in your mind some person or animal you care about. Remember a time they gave you a look that reminded you how much you love them. Feel the heartfelt connection you have with them. After about twenty seconds of this, slowly open your eyes. To many people's surprise, the Relaxation Breath can quickly and dramatically reduce a craving for a cigarette.

The final method to help you overcome the smoking habit is something I call the Smoker's Contract. This contract will help keep you motivated to use the smoking substitutes I've previously outlined. Basically, it consists of an agreement you make with yourself to gradually cut down the amount you smoke each day by three cigarettes until you've quit. For example, if you're a pack a day smoker, you'd write down that on Tuesday you can have seventeen cigarettes, on Wednesday, you can have fourteen cigarettes, and so on, until you reach zero. During the day you try to pace yourself so you don't smoke more than your allotted amount before you go to sleep. If, however, you decide to smoke any "extra" cigarettes on a given day, before smoking it, take out $2 and rip it to shreds. I mean it.

As you slowly cut down on how much you smoke, you'll occasionally face a choice between smoking an extra cigarette you want, ripping up $2, or doing one of the smoking substitutes. Given this choice, there's a good chance you'll try one of those methods. Yet, even if you rip up the $2, you're still keeping to your agreement with yourself. I guarantee that if you keep to the terms of the contract you make with yourself, you'll soon be smoke-free. I've helped hundreds of smokers quit using this method. Even if you don't think it'll work, it works. To make sure your Smoker's Contract works, make sure you write exactly what you plan to do on a single piece of paper. Your contract might look like the following:

I, Lucy, agree to the following contract regarding cigarettes:

On Tuesday, March 4, I can smoke up to seventeen cigarettes.

On Wednesday March 5, I can smoke up to fourteen cigarettes.

On Thursday March 6, I can smoke up to eleven cigarettes.

On Friday March 7, I can smoke up to eight cigarettes.

On Saturday March 8, I can smoke up to five cigarettes.

On Sunday March 9, I can smoke up to two cigarettes.

On Monday, March 10, I will be smoke-free.

For each "extra" cigarette I choose to smoke, I agree to rip up $2 BEFORE smoking it.

(Your signature)   (Today's Date)

When you do the contract, make sure you count out the correct amount of cigarettes you can smoke each day before you have to rip up money. Tell your friends that you're quitting so they can encourage you through the process and keep you accountable. Some people complain that they should be able to donate the $2 to charity, or give it to someone. Unfortunately, my experience has shown that this doesn't work. Ripping up $2 is painful, and it is the desire to avoid that pain that can motivate you to skip the cigarette and do something else instead. To deal with the discomfort of cutting down and eventually quitting cigarettes, you'll begin to rely on the smoking substitutes. Soon, these simple methods or ways of changing how you feel will be your new "friend." They'll help you to handle the stresses in life rather than sucking on cancer sticks. Before you know it, your friends and family will be congratulating you, you'll have more energy, and you'll feel proud of yourself. Don't put it off!

15: Lose Weight Permanently

The Accountability Contract

The verdict is in—diets don't work. If they did, one-third of all Americans wouldn't be obese. In one major study, people who dieted ended up gaining an average of three pounds over the long term every time they went on a diet. So if diets don't work, what does? It seems like every year there are many hot new theories of how to lose unwanted pounds. Some of these theories even work if you meticulously follow the program. Therein lies the rub. Not many people have the inclination to know exactly how many grams of protein versus carbohydrates to have at each meal. However, instead of counting grams, calories, or taking diet pills, there are three fundamentals that everyone agrees are helpful in order to lose weight. By providing you with a method for staying consistent with the fundamentals, you can slowly but surely lose weight.

There is no getting around the three fundamentals. You can't cheat your body—it knows what you're doing to it. The three are: consistent exercise, eating less foods with high fat or calories, and eating more foods that are good for you, such as fruits and vegetables. Most people know this, they just can't get themselves to do it consistently. Unfortunately, when it comes to losing weight, what really matters is what you do consistently. Starving yourself one week or exercising two hours a day for a few days will do you little good if you can't faithfully practice the fundamentals. That's why what's needed is a plan and motivational method to make sure you regularly carry out the three central tenets of effective weight management. Fortunately, I've found that there is a simple and effective way to get yourself to do the behaviors you know are good for you. I call it the Accountability Contract, or AC for short.

There are two simple theories that underlie why the AC works so well. First, people tend to do things to avoid immediate pain and/or gain immediate pleasure. This makes losing weight difficult since eating fatty or high caloric foods is immediately pleasurable, whereas exercise and cottage cheese are not. The second theory is that people will do a lot to avoid the embarrassment of breaking clearly stated promises to another human being. The Accountability Contract makes use of these two psychological principles to help people stay consistent with eating right and exercising regularly. In the AC, you make a contract with someone you know to exercise a certain amount each week, and eat certain foods and not others. Then, once a week, you go over your contract with your accountability partner and see how you did. That's it!

While the general concept behind the AC is simple, there are subtleties to it you need to know to increase its effectiveness. For example, when writing a contract, it's important to be realistic about what you can do. If you didn't exercise last week at all, but put down you'll exercise an hour a day this week, you'll likely fail. Instead, start slowly and build on your successes. For example, you might begin with a contract like the following:

I, Jonathan, agree to do the following for the week of February 12:

1. Exercise (brisk walking) three times this week, for a minimum of twenty minutes each time.

2. Avoid eating anything after 8:00 P.M.

3. Eat at least one piece of fruit per day, and one vegetable.

4. Avoid eating any potato chips, and donuts, and limit cookie intake to one per day.

For each violation of the above contract, I agree to rip up $2.

Signed, Jonathan Robinson

As you can see, in this contract, I agree to rip up $2 if I fail to keep any of my commitments. My experience with hundreds of people has shown that the desire to avoid ripping up $2 greatly helps motivate people to fulfill their contract. Since ripping up money is very

your thumb and press it deeply into a spot near your heel. Creep the thumb (alternately straightening and bending) like a "caterpillar walk" throughout each section of your foot. Use as much pressure as you can without creating discomfort. Make sure you eventually reach all parts of the foot: the heal, the ball, the sides, the toes, and the base of the toes. By the time you're done with one foot, the other foot will likely be crying out for its turn. Give it its due.

Once you're done with the feet, you can do your own hands if you have time. The hands are a bit harder to do than the feet because you can use both hands to massage a single foot, but only one hand is free to massage the other. Nevertheless, the healing and enjoyable sensation that results can be as wonderful as when you massaged your feet. As you practice this art, you'll find your hands growing stronger, which can lead to even better sensations down the road.

Reflexology can quickly relax and invigorate your entire body. Yet, sometimes it's helpful to know how to use acupressure to alleviate a *specific* problem. For a headache, there are two points that are especially useful. First, move your thumb close to your index finger. Notice that this creates a small mound by the base of your thumb. By firmly pushing your index finger into the mound of the opposite hand, you can often feel something that could be described as "electrical." Apply this pressure for twenty seconds. Then, proceed to apply the same pressure to the mound of the other hand for twenty seconds. These points will not only help you combat a headache, but also help reduce tension.

The second acupressure point to reduce the pain of a headache can be found at the base of your skull. Place your thumbs at the indentations on both sides of your spine—where your neck and head meet. Press or massage these points with your thumbs for ten seconds, then repeat after a few moments of rest. You'll likely feel relief in a short amount of time. These headache cures shouldn't be overused. If you get a lot of headaches, it's a sign that you're not taking good care of yourself. By doing foot and hand reflexology periodically, you'll likely reduce the amount of tension headaches you get in the first place.

For PMS, many women have found that massaging the point right between the eyebrows for half a minute is helpful. While doing this, make sure you breathe deeply, take a brief break, then repeat. Another helpful acupressure point for PMS and cramps is the mound area between the thumb and index finger as previously described for headaches.

A good rule of thumb is that if a point on your body feels sore or tender, it's probably a good idea to massage it. Since the body is symmetrical, if you massage a point on one side of your body, it's best to massage the same area on the other side of your body. If you have a friend or mate who would be willing to give you a shoulder, neck, or scalp massage in exchange for one in return, then you're in luck. The shoulders, neck, and scalp are also filled with acupressure points that can help balance the entire body. Be willing to explore. As you massage various points of your body, you'll soon learn what feels good. And if it feels good, it's likely to be good for you. Enjoy.

17: Clean and Revive Your Body

The Power of Fasting

Fasting is probably the oldest healing method known. Although not used extensively in the United States, it is popular as a healing modality on virtually every continent. During a fast, the eliminative organs of the body, such as the skin, lungs, liver, bowels, and kidney, become more active. Since the body isn't spending energy digesting food, it can direct all its energy to eliminating accumulated toxins. Even animals know about fasting. It's natural for sick animals to avoid food so that their full body energy can be directed toward healing. After a fast ranging from one to ten days, your body will be cleaner, stronger, less toxic, and healthier. In addition, you'll weigh less, and likely be less addicted to harmful foods.

If you have little or no experience with fasting, it's important to seek the medical advice of your chosen health care practitioner. They can recommend what would be best for you to try based on your current health and needs. When I first began fasting, I started out by drinking only fruit and vegetable juices for a full day. As I fasted for longer periods of time, I found out it's important to use an enema each day of fasting, along with other methods for stimulating one's skin and lungs. By getting plenty of exercise and fresh air, I was able to help clear my lungs of toxins, and by brushing my skin with a skin brush twice a day, I was able to eliminate dead skin. I also found that saunas were useful for increasing perspiration, and that drinking plenty of liquids was absolutely critical for speeding up the detoxification process.

Typically the first day of a fast is only slightly difficult. You may feel a bit nauseous, hungry, or weak for a few moments. Such signs only mean that you're detoxifying and that things are proceeding as they should. The second and third day of a fast tend to be a bit more uncomfortable. The detoxifying process accelerates. Surprisingly, after three days of fasting, it becomes much easier to go without food. Typically, a person loses their appetite, and becomes mentally, emotionally, physically, and spiritually revitalized. After several days of not having anything except juices and water, your body will be remarkably cleaner and less toxic. Longer fasts, however, must be done under the supervision of a doctor or other health-care practitioner familiar with the fasting process.

A general rule of thumb for creating health is that doing anything is better than doing nothing. Therefore, a one-day fast isn't ideal but it's a lot better than nothing. Many people choose to do a one-day fast once a week as a way of keeping weight off and keeping their body healthy. If you eat meat, especially red meat, you might consider doing a one-week meat fast. Although this isn't as powerful as a juice-only fast, it will give your body a slight rest from your usual diet. However long or frequently you fast, it's important to begin it with empty bowels and a good disposition.

When I ask most people why they don't fast, the typical response is that it's too hard. Nevertheless, it may be a lot easier than you think. Hunger pains only last a few minutes, and in most cases are not very intense. If you do have problems with hunger, make yourself a smoothie. Putting a banana in a blender full of apple juice and water (and vitamins in powder form—see chapter 9), can help you overcome hunger or feelings of weakness. The combination of fresh fruit, vitamins, minerals, and juice can give you a "zing" that makes you feel great. Since you won't have eaten in awhile, you'll be able to immediately feel the effect of the nutrients the smoothie is providing your body.

In order to avoid traumatizing your body, it's necessary to consider what to eat immediately before and after fasting. In general, you want to ease into a fast by avoiding meat for at least a couple of meals. The same is true when coming out of a fast. The longer the fast, the more important it is to ease back into eating solid foods. The best food to eat immediately following a fast is a little bit of fruit, because fruit is so easily digested. At a next meal, vegetables are good to eat. Since your body hasn't had any food for awhile, it can more easily absorb the nutrients of whatever you eat. If you've fasted for more than three days, it's wise to wait an equivalent number of days before you introduce hard to digest foods such as meat. The book *How to Keep Slim and Healthy with Juice Fasting* by Paavo Airola can provide you with more information about how to begin and end a fast.

If you are ill, it's a good idea to seek the advice of a trusted health care practitioner before deciding if it's appropriate to fast. Some diseases react well to fasting, whereas others do not. When not eating food, medicines can often have more effect than they normally would. If your medicine is in pill form, you might try to crush it with a spoon and dissolve it in a cup of tea so that you can drink your medication. It can also be a good idea to ask your doctor about the effects of fasting on any medicines you are currently taking.

Fasting is surely a shortcut to health. Besides saving you time, money, and calories, fasting revitalizes your entire state of health. Unfortunately, reading about fasting has no known benefits. You have to actually do a fast. Many people report that a fast is a great way to "start over" in life. It cleans the slate. Once your fast is over, you'll feel like the past is over and the future is brand new. You'll be in a more healthy position to seize the day.

18: Overcome a Bad Back

The Knack of Relaxing Your Back

Experts say that eight out of ten Americans will miss work at some point in their life due to a bad back. That's a lot of people. As someone who's had a bad back for awhile, I've tried it all. I've been to chiropractors, doctors, acupuncturists, physical therapists, surgeons, and massage therapists. After spending thousands of dollars, trying many remedies, and reading about a dozen books on the subject, I've concluded that the best way to handle a bad back is through some simple preventive strategies. Fortunately, the suggestions that follow are usually free or low cost. While they take a few minutes to do, they can save you from a lot of pain, trouble, and lost income due to not being able to work.

My first advice for people with occasional back problems is to avoid doing things that strain the back. For example, when lifting heavy objects, it's important to bend and lift with your legs instead of your back. It's especially dangerous to twist while lifting. Standing in one position for a long time is also stressful for the back. If you need to stand for awhile in one position, try to put one leg up on a footstool. Ideally, a footstool should be about a foot high. When driving, don't sit far back from the wheel. Stretching for the pedals decreases your low back curve—and increases back strain. Slumping in a chair is another way to reduce your natural low back curve and increase back strain. If possible, sit only in chairs where slumping is unlikely to happen. Finally, don't sleep on soft mattresses or couch cushions because of the additional strain they can cause.

In order to prevent back problems, there are many exercises that can be done to strengthen the surrounding muscles and make them more limber. Here are four of my favorites:

1) Stand in a comfortable position with your knees slightly bent, and place your hands in the low back area. Bend backwards (while supporting your low back with your hands), and hold for about forty-five seconds. Then slowly straighten.

2) Sit in a chair. Lean forward in your chair and lower your head to your knees and your hands to the floor. Stay in this relaxed position for two minutes.

3) Lie on your back with your knees bent and feet flat on the floor. As you breathe in, arch up your back muscles so that the small of your back is no longer on the floor, but your buttocks still are. As you exhale, press your lower back to the floor while tightening your abdomen and buttocks. Hold this position for five seconds, then repeat from the beginning. Do this five times.

4) While lying on your back with knees bent, cross your arms loosely over your chest and tuck your chin in. Curl the upper part of your body up off the floor, just enough to feel your abdomen muscles tighten. Hold for a count of five, then curl down. Repeat this as many times as you comfortably can. By strengthening your abdominal muscles, you can prevent many back problems.

If you would like more exercises to help strengthen and stretch your back area, send for a pamphlet called *Back Exercises for a Healthy Back* by Krames Communications. It can be ordered by calling (800) 333-3032. It costs $3.00 plus $1.95 shipping and handling.

Next, there is the area of back helping gadgets. I love gadgets, and I've noticed they're a lot cheaper than medical doctors or chiropractors. My favorite gadget for the money is a lumbar support pillow. You can get these in auto parts stores or Wal-Mart. Basically, they are cushions of various shapes and sizes that help support the natural curvature of the lower back. Most chairs and car seats are not designed for supporting this curve, which causes extra back strain. By having a lumbar cushion (or even a rolled up towel) give your lower back extra support, you'll find your back can feel comfortable for longer periods of time while sitting or driving.

Another great gadget you can buy is called a Ma Roller. The Ma Roller looks like a wooden rolling pin, but in the middle of it is an indentation for your spinal column. The way to use the Ma Roller is to lie down and place the roller under your lower back. Then, with your spine aligned with the indentation in the roller, slowly roll your body up and down the entire length of your back. The result is that the muscles on either side of your spine get a very deep level of massage. This helps to stimulate the acupuncture points along your spine, and loosen tight muscles. It can be painful if your muscles are tight, but ultimately it feels really good. A Ma Roller costs about $25, and can be found in Relax The Back stores throughout the country. For the store nearest you, call 1-800-290-2225, or order one through the mail by calling (805) 981-9964.

If and when you strain or injure your back, doctors recommend taking it easy for a couple of days. I have found that icing one's back can be especially helpful. A good way to "ice" your back is to buy a bag of frozen peas and place the bag in the area that feels injured. Applying heat to an injury is not a good idea since the pain is often caused by inflammation, and heat just makes it worse. Many drugstores also have gels of various kinds that can be put in the freezer and applied (over clothing) to an injured part of your body. I have found Motrin to be particularly effective in reducing pain and inflammation, or even better is the prescription medication Indomethacin.

If back problems persist, it's a good idea to see a doctor or chiropractor. But beware—the high-priced doctors I visited always said they would be able to help, yet rarely did. The best treatment for a bad back is prevention. Part of prevention is to avoid undue amounts of stress which can lead to chronic back and neck tension. In fact, one of the best-known back experts in the country, Dr. John Sarno, says that almost all back problems are due to stress, not to structural abnormalities. He recommends that people say certain affirmations that help make it clear that the problem is basically in one's head. I found his book, *Healing Back Pain: The Mind-Body Connection,* to be helpful and worth checking out if you have persistent back problems.

As with most health care concerns, a good defense is your best investment. By taking small, reasonable steps to prevent back strain, you can prevent costly long-term problems. As with most things in life, you get the best results from being consistent with whatever program you decide is right for you.

19: Effectively Handle Big Health Problems

The Skill of Surviving an Illness

Each year, tens of thousands of people die from less than life-threatening conditions in their homes and in hospitals. They die of minor infections that quickly get out of control. They die of fouled-up medical treatment. They die from not taking the right medications for their condition. In addition, many studies conclude that hundreds of thousands of people each year undergo surgery that was not necessary or even desirable. How can you prevent becoming one of these statistics? The more you know, the better off you'll be and the more likely you'll get the best treatment possible. To survive big health problems, you need to avoid passively doing whatever your doctor says, and instead take an active role in your own treatment program. By heeding the advice that follows, you can get better treatment, avoid costly and dangerous mistakes, and feel more in control while facing a fearful situation.

When facing a serious medical condition, the first thing to consider is getting good medical advice. The doctor you know may not be an expert in the condition you have. Ask friends, doctors, and family members for their recommendations. You can even look on the Internet for information on experts associated with your particular problem. Last year, when my dog starting having seizures, I was able to download a bunch of information that the local vets were not aware of. The information I gathered was very helpful in leading to a treatment that finally worked. In a similar way, you may want to check out chat rooms, newsgroups, or online health information resources, such as: www.mayohealth.org or www.intelihealth.coms. The more you know about the condition you have, the better your chances for success will be.

Once you've done your homework, your next step is to interview the top names or health care institutions you're considering for help. Be sure to bring all relevant information to the people you interview, such as angiograms, blood test results, MRIs, etc. It can also be helpful to have a list of questions to ask each of them. Below is a brief list of questions, but you can add your own. A good health care practitioner will not be put off by your sincere questions. The answers you receive can provide you with even more information about your condition and treatment options. In addition, by their demeanor, you'll gain important insight into whether or not they're the person you want to treat you.

Questions to ask your doctor or other health care provider:

1. What do you see as my treatment options, and why do you recommend one treatment over another?

2. How important is it to do something right away, as opposed to waiting and seeing how things develop?

3. What are the risks before, during treatment (such as during surgery), and after? What percentage of people die from this condition, and what percentage have a full recovery after treatment?

4. How painful will the treatment be? Are there medications that can safely reduce the pain?

5. How long will I be in the hospital? How long will it be until I can go back to work or do simple activities such as drive my car?

6. After treatment or surgery, will I need ongoing care such as a home health care nurse, exercise program, special diet, etc?

7. What can I do to best prepare myself for the treatment or surgery?

8. Are there any other specialists in this field you would recommend I see for another opinion?

Many people feel uncomfortable asking the last question in this list. They feel it's an insult to the doctor or practitioner they're talking to. Perhaps it is. Ask it anyway. There are a lot of incompetent doctors out there. When I was having severe back problems a couple of years ago, the first doctor I saw recommended I have several of my spinal discs fused together in an operation that was going to cost $50,000 and leave me hobbling for the rest of my life. Fortunately, the opinion I received from two other doctors was that three minutes of back exercises per day was appropriate for my condition. Now, three years later, my back seems fine. I feel sorry for people who don't seek out second opinions. In general, the more severe your condition or the proposed treatment, the more opinions you should seek.

Nowadays, there is an endless list of alternative treatments for almost every condition. People frequently make one of two mistakes when considering alternative treatments. The most common one is to not even consider them. The second most common mistake is to think they're the only thing that will work. Somewhere between these two extremes lies the truth. In general, studies reveal that several modes of treatment are likely to lead to better results than just a single mode of treatment. For example, women with breast cancer who have a mastectomy live longer than those who don't. But women who have a mastectomy and belong to a psychological support group do the best of all. Studies even reveal that when prayer is added to a treatment regime it significantly impacts the outcome in a positive way. Therefore, whenever possible, try alternative treatment methods in addition to Western medicine.

During severe illness, people are sometimes unable to communicate their treatment wishes. To avoid this problem, prepare in advance an Advance Directive or Durable Power of Attorney for Health Care Decisions. In simple language this means you make your wishes known to a trusted friend or family member regarding various medical treatments. In the event that a serious illness or injury leaves you too incapacitated to make your wishes known, the person you've selected will make decisions for you. This person should know your desires regarding life-saving measures such as artificial respirators, kidney dialysis, and other extreme measures.

In order to put someone in charge of your wishes if you're incapacitated, you need them to fill out a special form. You can ask your physician how to obtain such a form, or many stationary stores that carry business forms have them. Every person who is over eighteen should have both a Will and an Advance Directive. It's one of those things that people don't like to think about, but it's important. Make copies of each to give to your physician and family. In fact, after you update your Will and Advance Directive, ask your family members and friends about theirs. In case of an emergency or tragedy, such documents can make a bad situation a bit more tolerable. Without a Will or Advance Directive, emotional chaos can ensue for a long, long time.

Finally, make sure that once you receive appropriate treatment you don't let things slide with your aftercare. Not long ago, a friend of mine died of internal bleeding after a seemingly successful operation. Evidently, he didn't follow the doctor's orders regarding how to take care of himself after surgery. The relief from surgery can sometimes lead people to feel that they've "made it." Yet, very few people die in surgery. Most people die from complications after surgery or other forms of intense treatment. Therefore, make sure you're as diligent after your treatment as before. Continue to get up-to-date information on how to recover from your condition, and use alternative health care methods if you deem them helpful.

The most important thing to know when facing a serious health condition is that you have choices. The more you know, the better the decisions you can make. In the face of fear, some people let their emotions lead them to passively accept whatever the first expert recommends. That's the worst thing you can do. No one cares as much about your condition as you. Read up on your condition, ask questions, know your options. Besides helping you get the best care possible, your active participation in your treatment will help you feel more in control and better able to recover.

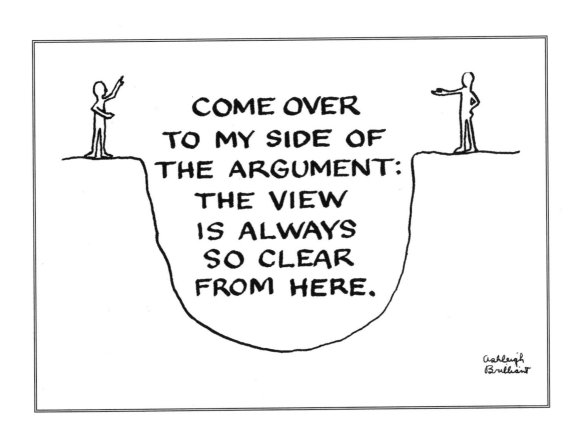

Better Relationships

To a large extent, our lives are successful or not depending on the quality of our relationships. That's because whatever we might want in life—love, money, spiritual growth, respect—is achieved through our interactions with people. However, despite the obvious importance of relationships, most of us are not trained in the skills of having better, deeper, or more harmonious connections with people. Yet even business schools are now starting to see the importance of such training. Recently, Harvard Business School did a study of the importance of "people skills" in business. After giving their M.B.A. graduates some tests to separate the students who had "good people skills" from those who did not, they followed these two groups of graduates for five years to see how they fared. They found that after five years, the graduates who ranked in the top 10 percent of the class in "people skills" were making 85 percent more money than the bottom 10 percent of the class in people skills! The researcher's conclusion was that skills in relating to people were just as important as technical training and education in making a good income.

Some folks think you are either born with the ability to get along well with people, or you're not. This is not true. In my own case, I was a painfully shy child and teenager. As a young teen, I had no friends and I rarely spoke. It was only after reading books such as *How to Win Friends and Influence People* that I learned how to make friends. As I learned these skills, it was like exploring a whole new world. Fortunately, although people are very complex, the skills needed to know how to be successful in relationships are very teachable. In this section, you'll learn what really makes human beings tick, how to deal with difficult people, how to "win people over," and how to develop mutually satisfying business and personal relationships.

20: Solve Problems Without Bruising Egos

The Art of Effective Compromise

Most people do everything wrong when trying to solve a problem with someone else. They try to imitate a lawyer prosecuting a witness, showing the other person all the ways their position is faulty. In a phrase, they play the "blame game." Unfortunately, blame never works. But there is an easy method that *does* work. Once you learn it, you'll be amazed at how easily and quickly you can solve even entrenched problems once you know the right methods.

The first step in any conflict is to bolster the ego of the person you're dealing with. This is exactly the opposite of what most people do. Most people present evidence showing how wrong someone else is, hoping that this will change their mind. Of course, this never works—the other person just gets more defensive. This happens because inside everyone's brain is a little-known gland called a "blame detector" which shuts off our ear canals whenever we sense we're being told we are wrong. When we feel blamed, it lessens our self-esteem, and in an attempt to "save face," we refuse to admit there is *anything* to what someone else is saying. That's why it's much better to do the exact opposite—tell the person you're dealing with what you like about him or her. If there is something valuable in their plan or approach to a problem, tell them that as well. That will make them more receptive to what *you* have to say. Since you've complimented them and shown you've listened to their ideas, they will think you're intelligent, and will then feel obligated to listen to you.

Once you've bolstered the ego of the other person, explain precisely what you see the problem as, and what you hope to achieve by coming to an effective compromise. For example, let's say a man named Bob employs a woman named Cheryl who is chronically late. Bob might say, "Cheryl, I appreciate how efficient you've been in getting the reports done. You're fast and effective at getting a lot done in a little time. I've also noticed that you were late to work twice this past week, and that worries me. I'd like to figure out a way to handle this problem so that both you and I can continue to feel respected and work well together." When Bob states what he hopes to achieve from an effective compromise, he explains the ultimate result he would like, not his preferred solution. Had Bob said, "I want you to be on time from now on," Cheryl would have probably felt resentful and unheard. But because Bob stated what he ultimately wants, namely to feel respected and work well together, Cheryl would likely be more receptive to what Bob has to say.

Recently, I was booked by an organization to stay at a hotel near where I was to speak. When I went to check in at the desk, the clerk said they had no record of my reservation, and that they had no vacancies. Immediately I told the clerk he must be mistaken, but my curt words resulted in him just getting defensive. So, I changed strategies. I told him, "I apologize for my abruptness. I know employees at this hotel are well trained, and I'm sure that if you couldn't find a reservation for me, then it must not be in the computer." I went on to say, "From past experience I know how dedicated you folks are to working things out, so I wonder if you have any ideas as to what could be done." He said he'd talk to his boss, and upon his return said, "We have a room on the fourth floor, will that be okay?" I don't know how this room "magically" appeared, and I didn't really care. All I cared about was the fact that the problem was resolved.

In the previous example, I did something very few people do. Once my initial remark didn't work, I changed strategies. When a communication doesn't work, many people simply say the same thing again—only louder. Not a good move. Instead of ranting and complaining, I indirectly complimented the clerk. Then I took the final step in successful problem solving: I asked him if he had any ideas as to how *he* might solve the problem at hand. Asking people for *their* solutions is much better than telling them yours—at least initially. When you ask someone for their ideas, it shows respect. They are much more likely to listen to you once you've listened to them.

If the person or people you're talking to comes up with a good solution, tell them you love the idea. If their ideas are not acceptable, or if they don't have any ideas, ask them, "Would you be willing to hear a couple of ideas I have which might work better for both of us?" That's a great question. Since you've already listened to them, they'll feel obligated to listen to your solutions. Once several ideas are out on the table, it's just a matter of negotiating and compromising your way to an acceptable conclusion.

Sometimes people are reluctant to agree to a compromise because they fear they'll have to commit to it for a long time. Instead, why not suggest that you try a specific compromise for a set time, say a week or a month? This will make it easier to move forward, especially if you reassure the person you're dealing with that if after a month it isn't working to their satisfaction, you'd be willing to try something else. Even many entrenched problems can be remedied through being willing to try various short-term solutions and seeing what works. If you can avoid bruising the ego of the person you're talking to, you'll find it relatively easy to come up with workable solutions. Telling people what you like about them, explaining the ultimate result you hope to achieve, asking them for their solutions first, and trying short-term compromises are all tools to help efficiently solve problems. Once you get good at these skills, you'll have a new problem: a lot more people wanting to work with you or spend time with you. Some problems are worth having.

21: Make a Relationship Special

The Joy of Peak Moments

Why do people travel halfway around the world to visit a place such as Disneyland, pay $40 to get in, and stand in line for an hour for a three-minute ride? Because, as human beings, we crave peak moments. The desire for an intense, special, extraordinary experience is one of our deepest desires. That's one of the major reasons why we like sex, falling in love, winning a big game, and weddings. Yet peak moments need not be reserved for such major events. You can learn to create them in daily life with people you care about. Once you learn the skill of creating special times for other people, your relationships will never be the same. People will want to know you, do business with you, and even marry you because you know how to create a sense of aliveness wherever you are. There are four key concepts that can help you create more peak moments with your friends, mate, coworkers, and family.

1) This is perhaps the most obvious, but also the most difficult: make extraordinary times with people you care about a *priority* in your life. If I said "I'll give you $50,000 if you can create a peak moment with your mate or coworker this month," could you do it? I bet you could. Simply by having enough motivation, you'd find a way. After all, you've shared special moments with people before. How'd you do it? You somehow created a special event, setting, or mood that had an aura of uniqueness to it. Well, I can't give you fifty grand to do it

again. However, if you make this idea a priority in your life, the rewards you receive will be worth more than just money.

Many years ago, I used to visit elder care facilities. When I would talk to the people about their lives, they would often convey a special moment they remembered, such as kissing their mate under a waterfall or a romantic dinner shared under the stars. When I'd ask them to convey some of their advice and wisdom to me, the most frequent theme was the importance of really "going for it" in life. One nintey-year-old woman named Vye pleaded with me, "Don't get lost in all the trivial, mundane stuff in life. Remember to create magic times you'll remember with the people you love." Great advice from a very wise woman.

2) Be fully yourself. What does that mean? It means saying what you really think and feel, and doing what you really want to do. Children are naturally fully themselves, and that's one reason why they're so easy to love. In this age of mediocrity, machines, and mechanical behavior, people thirst for authenticity and aliveness. One way to tap into being fully yourself is to ask the question, "How would I be different if I weren't inhibited by fear or other people's opinions of me?" Would you be more honest, more outrageous, or more unusual? Most people would.

When I was in high school, my best friend Brian decided he was going to be fully himself. He began wearing unusual clothes that he liked, rather than what was currently "in." He would say whatever was on his mind, such as his true opinion of an arrogant teacher or a snobbish girl. He even started playing his favorite game, *mahjong,* right in the middle of the main lunch hangout. Within two months, he went from being an unknown kid to the most popular student on campus. When Brian was around, there was always laughter, unpredictability, and aliveness. It was wonderful. He showed me that stepping beyond one's fear could be a magnetic force that powerfully attracts people.

3) Be willing to plan special moments. Many peak moments simply come from being spontaneous, or being fully yourself. Many don't. Being willing to carefully plan such experiences will give you an added approach to making them happen. So how can you create such an experience for someone you care about? The key is to know what someone else would greatly enjoy. Does he or she like surprises, such as a birthday party or a trip to a beautiful spot in nature? Does he or she like gifts, such as flowers or perhaps a favorite meal delivered at home? By knowing a person, you should be able to make a good guess as to what would be appreciated. If you're planning a peak moment for someone you don't know very well, ask his or her friends what they think would be greatly enjoyed.

A good rule of thumb is that the more unique an experience is, the more it will be remembered. Having flowers delivered to your office is nice, but if the person delivering the flowers breaks out in a song of love or congratulations, you're more likely to remember it. One of the more memorable times in my life was when, for my birthday, a friend rented weather balloons filled with helium to send me flying skywards in a lawn chair. Such experiences are not easily forgotten.

4) In order to powerfully affect someone, tell the person you're sharing a special moment with what he or she means to you. Most people are practically starving to hear words of appreciation. We all want to be valued and acknowledged, but there are few forums for doing so in today's busy culture. At the same birthday as the one with the helium balloons, my friends each shared a story about how I had positively impacted their lives. It was very powerful for me to hear how I had touched them. More than the helium balloons and lawn chair, I'll always remember how I felt when friends expressed their feelings about me.

With the four keys I've described here, you can unlock the doors to many magical experiences. Creating peak moments for those you care about is not only fun and rewarding, but it's also contagious. Soon, you may find your mate, friends, and coworkers creating such experiences for you.

22: Easily Handle Difficult People

Turning Tigers Into Pussycats

Whether on the job or in one's personal life, we all have to deal with "difficult" people on occasion. The most troublesome people to deal with are those that fly off the handle at the smallest problem. I call these people "tigers" because they can be quick and deadly. Yet. there are also other types of difficult folks we have to contend with. There are the gossipers, the backstabbers, and the naggers. In order to create successful relationships we need to know how to effectively handle people when they go into these modes of operation. The sad truth is that most people's normal or habitual way of handling difficult people—getting angry at them or staying silent—tends to be like putting gasoline on a fire. It simply doesn't work. Still, there are simple strategies for turning tigers into pussycats and transforming backstabbers, gossipers, and naggers into sincere, honest human beings.

The first step in dealing with any difficult person is to hear what he or she has to say, and to acknowledge their current reality. Acknowledging their reality does not mean you agree with him or her, it just means you understand their feelings and what they're trying to say. For example, let's say your boss, Bob, steps into your office and yells, "Where the hell is the McKenzie report? I told you I wanted it on my desk by noon. I'm sick and tired of always having to wait for you to get things done on time!" Your recollection is that the report wasn't due for another week, and that you *always* have things done on time. However, if you say that, it will just escalate his anger. Therefore, you need to first acknowledge his feelings by saying something like, "I see you're upset about not having the report. I can understand that it would be frustrating to expect the report and then have to wait around for it."

Bob will either immediately calm down once you acknowledge his experience, or he'll blurt out a bit more anger. If he is still angry, that means he needs to have his reality acknowledged again. By doing this, he'll eventually calm down. Once he's vented what he needs to say, and you've acknowledged his reality (even if it's totally bogus), then you have created an opening where he can actually hear what *you* have to say. If you try to explain your position to him beforehand, his ear canals will be totally closed (anger does that to people). So what should you say? The best thing to do with any type of difficult person is to ask them questions to help clarify their intentions and what they want. In the case of Bob, you might say, "I know you're upset, but what do you think would be best to do considering that the report isn't done?" You may have to ask a question like this several times before they answer. Basically, by asking such a question, you're putting the problem back in Bob's lap, and giving him control over the situation.

Asking questions that clarify what a person wants is a great way to avoid further difficulties. It takes two to have an argument, and if you simply ask questions, there can be no disagreement. By listening to a tiger and then redirecting his anger toward what he really wants, you can avoid being the ongoing target of his or her wrath. If what he or she wants is not possible for you to give (such as a report being done when it obviously isn't done), you can put the problem back into their lap again by asking, "Since the report isn't done now, how do you think we should handle it from here?" Once again, by asking another question, you give them control and redirect their anger toward dealing with the reality of the situation.

When dealing with naggers, it's best to treat them the same way you would a tiger. Simply listen to their tale of woe, acknowledge their reality, then ask them a question that forces them to come up with creative solutions. For example, if Sharon is always nagging you about how she has too much work and she needs more time off, listen and acknowledge her stress. Then ask, "Since your job seems to always have a lot of stress and has certain hours, what do you think can be done differently to better handle it?" Perhaps Sharon's answer will involve you changing how *you* do something. If it's a good idea, use it. If it's an unworkable idea, simply say, "I'm afraid I can't do that particular suggestion. Are there any other ideas you have for how to better handle this problem?" Such an approach will usually lead to a solution, or at least end the nagging.

While naggers and tigers are up front about their displeasure, gossips and backstabbers are harder to deal with because they go behind your back. However, eventually you will hear something that confirms your suspicions about what they're doing. When that happens, you need to take action or they'll consider you a doormat. If you fail to stand up to their behind-the-back exploits, they'll likely keep trying to damage your reputation. The primary way to deal with such people is to expose their true intentions. The simplest manner to help reveal their intentions is to ask questions that make them accountable for their actions. For instance, if you hear that Mary said something negative about how you managed a project, you can say, "Mary, I heard from Joe that you didn't think I managed the new filing project very well. I'm wondering why you didn't come to me about that? What were you trying to accomplish?"

Mary is likely to respond in one of three different ways: apologize for what she did, deny that she said what she is accused of, or avoid talking about it with you. If she apologizes, you can ask that she clear things up with Joe. Even if she denies or avoids the subject, she is on notice that you are not a doormat. Your confronting her by asking a question that reveals her true intentions will make it less likely she will pick on you in the future. After all, backstabbers and gossips like to work in the dark. When they learn that they can't get away with anything with you, they will likely pick on someone else.

When a backstabber or gossip denies they said or did something, you can further confront him or her by saying something like the following: "Joe expressed concern to me about the filing project, and said that you had mentioned it was handled poorly. Would you mind both of us talking with Joe to clear up any misunderstandings about how it's going?" If your backstabbing coworker has nothing to hide, then he or she won't mind talking it out. If they do have something to hide, they may come up with some excuse to avoid "talking it out." At that point you can say, "Because you said (whatever they said), this is what happened. Was that your intention?" By asking such pointed questions, you show that you will not tolerate this type of behavior.

Unfortunately, tigers, gossips, backstabbers and naggers are here to stay. But by knowing effective strategies for handling such people, you can largely avoid having to deal with their negative habits. Once difficult people see you are unwilling to fall into their traps, they will either turn into pussycats, or turn their attention toward more unsuspecting folks. Either way, you'll save yourself a lot of time and aggravation by knowing how to handle them effectively.

23: How to Create Lifelong Friends and Business Contacts

The Power of Deliberate Kindness

Armed with the secret information I am about to reveal to you, you will soon have incredible power in making friends and business contacts. Since these human technologies are so powerful, I must first give you some warnings as to how to use them. Please don't use the ideas I'm about to divulge as a way to manipulate people. If you do, people will eventually see through your charade. Instead, consider these tools for connecting with people as a way to extend your good, caring intentions. If you use these methods with good intentions, you and the people you connect with will be amply rewarded.

The first key to making lifelong friends and business contacts is to know exactly what people really want. In my opinion, each human being wants to be respected as a unique and worthy individual. There are several ways to show people how much you value them, but perhaps the easiest is to simply listen to them with great respect and empathy. We all want to be thought of as interesting and unique, so when someone seems fascinated by what we have to say, it affirms our sense of worth. I don't suggest you fake being fascinated by others; I suggest you really *become* fascinated by what each person you meet has to say. Since good listeners are so rare, as you show respect and admiration for the person you're with, you'll become trusted and admired.

In today's fast-paced world, there's good news and bad news when it comes to making lifelong friends and business contacts. The bad news is that we're all so distracted with so much to do, it's harder than ever to nourish good connections. The good news is that we're all so busy that simple acts of kindness stand out like a great triumph of the human spirit. Someone once said that the best way to make a friend is to *be* a friend. It could also be said that the best way to make a loyal customer is to show them you *are* a friend. When friends or customers are convinced you really care about them, they'll become willing to go the extra mile for you. Since both personal and professional success depend on how you get along with people, knowing how to turn someone into a friend can change your life.

A second specific strategy for connecting at a deeper level with people is to simply tell them directly how much you appreciate them. Sincere, heartfelt compliments don't cost you anything, yet they can have a major impact on your friends and coworkers just because they're so rare. I have found that complimentary letters, preferably written by hand, are even more powerful. The simple act of writing a thank you note for something a friend has done for you can have major impact. In addition, brief letters of congratulations to others for important milestones in their life can also make a lasting impression. I remember that when I was on my first national television show, my friend Paul wrote a letter of congratulations, expressing how proud he was of me. Somehow, his words of congratulations put our friendship in a different class than all my other friendships. It showed he was attentive to my life, and that he really cared. I've never forgotten it, and our friendship is still strong to this day.

The man who is considered the world's greatest salesman, according to the *Guinness Book of World Records*, credits much of his success to consistently sending his past customers a postcard each month that says something like, "I appreciate you. Have a Happy Thanksgiving" (or whatever holiday is coming up). Although his cards, and even his *signature* are computer generated, he has found that people love to hear his simple messages of appreciation. By consistently sending his past customers such communications, he noticed that his referral rate for new customers went through the roof. If a clearly insincere message can have such an impact, just imagine how powerful your sincerely written letters of appreciation can have on your friends, business contacts, and coworkers.

Along with letters showing you care, small gifts can help to demonstrate your valuation and gratitude for the people in your life. Years ago I used to work at a place in which the receptionist was always doing helpful things for me and the other employees. Finally, as a token of my appreciation, I bought her some flowers. Upon giving them to her, she began to cry. She said, "I've worked here for seventeen years and no one has ever given me flowers." It was a beautiful experience for me to see how moved she was by my simple act of kindness. As time passed, I noticed she began to do extra favors for me, and our level of connection deepened. When I made a mistake at work, she was the first to stand up for me. Nowadays, I try to remember that small gifts are not small to the people who receive them. Heartfelt acts of kindness are long remembered.

Lastly, to make lifelong friends and business contacts, it's necessary to keep a Rolodex or electronic file of addresses and phone numbers of people you connect with. Some executives have said that their Rolodex is their most important asset. People like to do business with people they know and like, and if you have a sizeable mailing list, you have the equivalent of money in the bank. A friend of mine found a high-paying job simply by sending a letter describing what he was looking for to the 300 friends and business contacts on his mailing list. Another friend of mine found his mate through a similar process. No matter what you're looking for, someone you know can likely help you to find it. Studies show that most mate and high-paying jobs are found through networking. By keeping a current mailing list of people you know, and using it when you need to, you can create seemingly magical results in your life.

The suggestions I've made here are not new or surprising. But their consistent implementation are. We live in a highly depersonalized world. Acts of kindness, words of gratitude, and small gifts of appreciation can make a lasting impression on the people you interact with. Simply put, when you invest in the people around you, people will invest in you. Before you get busy with the next thing to do in your life, ask yourself, "How can I begin to implement these ideas on a somewhat consistent basis?" Perhaps you can create a calendar of when your friend's and coworker's birthdays are, or a system of reminding you to write letters of appreciation on occasion. Try it as an experiment. You'll be amazed at how your acts of generosity boomerang back to you.

24: Get Others to Really Hear You

How to Talk to an Alien

In the movie, *Close Encounters of the Third Kind,* scientists communicate with an alien culture through the use of musical notes. While music is not our primary way to communicate, in the movie it was used as a form of conveying information that the aliens could understand. In a similar way, we need to learn to talk in ways that members of species far different from us, such as the opposite sex, can readily understand. Even though most of us speak English, it is often very difficult to really understand others—or for them to understand you. Fortunately, there is a little-known language for talking to "aliens," such as your mate or boss, that they will easily grasp. It is the language of shared experience, that is, metaphors. The great communicators throughout history, from Jesus Christ to Oprah Winfrey, have all learned the magic of speaking in analogies and metaphors. Fortunately, learning to speak this way is a skill that can be easily learned. Once you know the basic technique, you'll be amazed at how much more quickly and effectively you can get across what you want to say.

Metaphors are simple phrases that help us understand an experience by linking it to something we're already familiar with. For example, when someone says, "My work is like a war zone," it helps us to quickly grasp what their situation is like. By using metaphors when you talk to others, you can help them better understand what you have to say. In addition, by making the metaphors specific to the person you're talking to, you can powerfully engage them in what you're hoping to convey. When Jesus the told fishermen, "I can make you fishers of men," he was speaking their language, and they responded. When you speak the language your mate, employees, or boss understands, each will respond. In fact, if they don't seem to be really hearing you, it means you probably are not speaking their language and it's time to try something else.

To learn this skill, it's helpful to decide in one or two sentences the basic message you would like to convey to someone. For instance, if you want to convince a customer to buy your computer software, you could ask yourself, "Why should this person switch to my software as opposed to the one he's been using?" Let's say your answer is that, in the long run, it will save him the time and aggravation of trying to continually upgrade his old software. Then ask yourself, "When has this person ever experienced a waste of time that greatly aggravated him?" If you know of a specific incident, such as the time he bought some widgets from another company for less money, but it ended up not working out well, then you can use this as a metaphor. You might say, "Mr. Smith, trying to stay with your old software is like you trying to buy those widgets for less money than ours. It might seem to save you time in the short term, but in the long term it'll just be a lot of aggravation and a waste of time."

When you use a metaphor that incorporates a person's own experience from the past, it's especially powerful. Of course, you often won't know a person's past experience well enough to tailor a metaphor that fits the current situation. However, you *can* come up with generic metaphors that will work almost as well. For example, in the previous example, you could have said, "Trying to keep using your old software is like trying to keep your old car running once it's begun breaking down regularly. After awhile, you realize it's just not worth taking it to the shop every month, and you're better off simply getting a new one."

To come up with useful analogies and metaphors, you can ask yourself the question, "When has this person ever experienced something akin to what I'm trying to convey?" This question also works when you want to create a metaphor to convey your feelings to an intimate partner. For instance, if your mate occasionally criticizes you, and they really haven't "gotten" how much this bothers you, you might want to create a metaphor to describe how much it annoys you. You could say, "When you tell me I'm a bad cook, I feel like I've been kicked in the groin." Of course, if you know your mate has also been hurt by harsh criticism, you can use an example from his or her specific past. You might say, "When you tell me in a harsh manner that I'm bad at something, it makes me feel like how you felt when (your ex-mate) Lee abandoned you in your time of need."

To help you do this, here's a simple three-step process to get you started:

1. Decide in a sentence or two what you're feeling or basically what you want to convey.

2. Ask yourself, "When has the person I want to communicate with ever had a similar experience?" If you aren't aware of similar past experiences they've had, ask yourself, "What is this experience I'm having akin to?" If possible, make a list of such experiences.

3. Choose one of those experiences and say, "When (briefly describe the situation) happens, it's like (briefly mention the corresponding situation)." Example: When you harshly criticize me, I feel like I'm a baby being screamed at by a drunken parent.

If you can create metaphors that effectively communicate your pain, or help people get in touch with the pain they're likely to feel if they don't change, you'll find them intently listening to you. In addition, if you can metaphorically communicate the *pleasure* they'll feel by doing what you suggest, they'll be all ears. The important thing is to speak in pictures, experiences, and phrases that emotionally grab people. Although we think of ourselves as very rational creatures, we mostly act based on what emotionally affects us. As you learn to speak to your mate, your friends, your customers, or your boss in ways they can relate to, you'll notice that the quality of their listening seems to take off. When people really feel heard, magic happens.

25: Give People What They Want

The Key to Harmonious Relationships

I used to have a housemate who would often leave her dirty dishes in the sink. Whenever she did this, I took it as a personal insult that she didn't respect me. One day I confronted her about this. She responded, "What do you mean I don't respect you? *You're* the one who doesn't respect me!" I was flabbergasted. I pointed out that I often washed her dishes without her even asking. She shot back, "That's exactly what I mean. You don't let me do my dishes when I want. You don't trust that I'll eventually do them. Instead, you make me feel guilty by doing them before I get to them." We had a long discussion about this and discovered that I had a "rule" or hidden expectation that a person should always do their dishes immediately after using them. On the other hand, she had a rule that a person should be allowed to clean their dishes whenever was a good time for them to do so. When two people secretly have different rules as to how things should be done, problems ensue. When two people have similar rules, or agreed-upon rules, harmony happens.

The great motivational speaker and author, Tony Robbins, defines rules as the standards a person has about what is needed in order to feel good about something. For example, how much time is okay for you to wait on hold on the phone before you get help? For some people, the answer is five seconds, for others it's fifty minutes. Those are very different rules. If your partner has a rule or expectation that they can keep you on hold for "a few minutes," and you have a rule that says "a few seconds," you're going to have problems. The same is true in business. I've waited on hold when calling some businesses for ten minutes, after which I normally hang up and never call them again. Obviously, their rules about the importance of "customer service" are different than mine. By knowing the most important rules of your partner, your boss, and your customers, you can create harmony and goodwill in your important relationships. When you fail to know this information, you can find yourself in a constant sea of problems.

It could be said that every upset between people is really a difference of opinion as to the "proper" way to do things. When we have a rule that is not respected by our partner, boss, or a particular business, we feel hurt. We think that *our* standards are the right ones, while *their* way of doing things is wrong. Blame sets in. However, what's really going on is that people have different standards or rules, and when they don't communicate them clearly, their rules often get violated. For example, I have a rule that says "When a business says something will be done on a certain date, it better be done on that date or I won't do business with them again." On the other hand, most businesses (in my experience) have a rule that says, "When we give a customer a date that the job will be done, that is our most optimistic assessment of when it might get done." With different rules like these, I've had a lot of upset in the past, and many businesses have lost me as a customer.

So, in order to create more success in relationships, the first step is to clearly define and communicate your rules to the appropriate people in your life. For example, nowadays when I need something done by a business, I tell them "Whatever date you tell me it'll be done, I expect it to be done by then. If it isn't, I'd like a 10 percent discount each day that it's late." Some businesses have balked at my "rule" while others have been fine with it. Obviously, I do business with the ones that can live by my rules. The way to define your own rules is to answer the question, "What does it take or what has to happen in order for me to feel good about...?" (Fill in the appropriate situation, such as "doing business with X company" or "our marriage.") To find out someone else's rules, you can ask them the same question. For example, you can ask, "What does it take or what has to happen in order for you to feel good about how we handle the money issues in our relationship?" (or whatever the situation you want to find out about).

Once you know your rules regarding a sensitive topic, it's a good idea to communicate them to the appropriate people. That way, they will not have to be psychic in order to give you what you want. In addition, if they don't want to play by the same rules, it's better to know that sooner rather than later. By asking your partner or people you do business with about what they need to feel satisfied, you can become much more efficient in gaining their goodwill. It does no good to bargain endlessly with your employees or customers over money when what they're really concerned about is something else. This is a common mistake. We tend to think that everyone has the same concerns, expectations, or rules that we do—like my housemate who had a different rule than I regarding dishwashing. Yet by asking questions such as, "What is most important to you here?" or "What would demonstrate my commitment to doing a great job for you?", you can find out information that is priceless.

It's important to bring up the subject of rules in a way that will make the other person receptive to a discussion. Whether you're wanting to clarify the rules of your partner or your customers, you can say something like the following: "I really value our connection, and I want to make sure we each get our needs met in a way that feels good for both of us. To help you and me establish a good long-term relationship, I think it would be helpful if you knew a couple of specific things about what I *most* appreciate, and what I have a difficult time with. I would also like to know what's most important to you, and what really bothers you so I can better satisfy your needs. For me, when it comes to the area of being on time (or whatever issue you want to bring up), I think you should know that I'm a bit of a stickler. I feel hurt when people are late, and I really appreciate it when people are on time. In order for you to feel good about me, what are your rules or expectations regarding being on time?"

Most people appreciate straightforward, honest communication such as this. It shows you really care and want to work things out. Whenever you spot a problem area with someone, assume you each have different rules, and try to get clarity as to exactly what rules each of you have. Once again, in order to find out someone else's rules ask, "In order for you to feel good about ____, what has to happen?" They might have a list of things. Pay careful attention. If some of their rules are in obvious conflict with your own, you may have to compromise, or recognize that you can't work together. (For more about this, see chapter 20.) Still, the biggest problems tend to occur when people are simply unaware of each other's rules, and end up violating them without even realizing it. Don't allow this to happen to you. Reveal your rules to others and ask others about what they most need or want from you. You'll soon notice how much better your relationships are.

26: Become Friendly with Strangers

The Art of Schmoozing and Mingling

Schmoozing is the art of getting people on your side. Whether you're wanting a date with someone you just met or the sale of a potential customer, you need to know how to schmooze if you don't want to lose. Some people think of schmoozing as a form of manipulation, and in a way they're right. But it's a "manipulation" to help someone else feel good. By knowing what makes people tick, you can quickly build rapport with them, gain their trust, and get them to like you. As you master some of the tricks of schmoozing, you'll notice that you'll become more successful in various areas of your life, both personal and professional.

The first thing to know about schmoozing is that people like it. We all want to be treated as special, and schmoozing is really the art of making people feel special. Of course, you can help people feel good about themselves just by carefully listening to them, giving them sincere compliments, and so on. An even more effective way to show people you care is to prepare something beforehand. There are three powerful ways to do this, known as the Gift, the Surprise, and the Secret Connection Schmooze.

In the Gift Schmooze, before going to meet someone, you buy them a small, appropriate gift. The simple act of giving someone a gift, even if they don't love it, shows that you cared enough to think of them beforehand. In a way, it doesn't much matter what you buy because anything you bring will be appreciated. A helpful resource for finding the perfect gift is a book appropriately titled *Finding the Perfect Gift* by Hullana and Preson. A few things I've brought people are boxes of chocolate candies, flowers, bottles of wine, and even lottery tickets. If you know a little about the person you're going to meet, you can buy something specifically right for them. Recently, I bought a national TV producer a box of her favorite type of candy. Not surprisingly, after the show she told me, "I'm going to do my best to get you back on the show again." Not bad for a $12 investment.

The Surprise Schmooze is one of my personal favorites because it's so much fun to do, and it has so much impact on the person who receives it. To create a Surprise Schmooze, before meeting the one to be schmoozed, ask yourself, "What could I do to have a surprise set up prior to our meeting?" The possibilities are endless, ranging from the simple to the Olympic. You could set it up so that the fortune cookie he gets at the restaurant you dine at has his name and a personalized prediction inside. You could get a few people who know this person to say (or write) nice things about him, and deliver the tape or letters personally at your meeting. Or you could simply personalize a gift, such as create a coffee mug with their picture on it, or a set of pens with their name engraved on it. Since such acts of caring are so rare, you'll stand out like a giant in a kindergarten class.

The Secret Connection Schmooze is simple, but it can also have terrific impact. To make use of this method, it helps to know a little bit about what's important to the person you're about to meet. Often, you can ask their employees, friends, coworkers, or family for this "secret" information. Simply call up someone who knows the person and ask, "What are they passionate about?" or "What do they love to do?" Then come prepared with a comment, story, article, or some information about their favorite topic. When you do this, you'll notice an instant connection.

When I wrote my book *The Experience of God* I needed to get interviews with famous spiritual leaders ranging from the Dalai Lama to the late Mother Teresa. To help me on my quest, before approaching such famous people, I'd do my homework. I'd find out specific things they liked, such as their favorite author or type of flower. When I wrote to them, I'd often include a comment about this "inside" information. When people ask me how I managed to interview forty of the best-known spiritual authors and leaders, I tell them, "With the power of my mind, I was able to create a secret connection with these people." Well, now you know my secret, and it's one you can also use with the "power" of *your* mind.

The Art of Mingling

Mingling is different than schmoozing in that a "schmooze" takes place between two people, whereas mingling is something that happens in groups. Yet, like schmoozing, the ability to mingle effectively can make a big difference in both your personal and business life. It's important to know that good minglers are not just born. With practice you can learn to feel more comfortable at mingling. And I've got three methods, the Compliment, the Honest technique, and the Question method, that can help you master the art of mingling.

The Compliment Mingle is just what it sounds like. When entering a group, such as at a cocktail party, compliment one of the people there, or even the entire group. For example, you might say, "There was so much laughing going on over here that I just had to see why you're having such a good time. What have you been talking about?" When directing your compliment to a specific person, you might choose to comment on an unusual article of clothing they're wearing. For example, you could say, "I couldn't help but notice how beautiful your earrings are. Where did you find something so unique?" Once you've made a compliment and asked a related question, you've completed the hardest part of mingling—breaking in. You're now ready for the Question Mingle.

The Question Mingle can be used to break into a group or to keep a conversation going. By asking questions, you indicate your interest and get people to talk about themselves. Fortunately, people love talking about themselves. Some of my favorite questions to ask when I enter a group or once I'm already in a group are:

1) So what do you think would help solve the current problem we have in… (briefly mention the current "crisis" in the news; people love to give their opinion about such stuff).

2) I'm doing a little survey on what book, besides the Bible, people think has been the most influential book ever written. What's your choice and why do you choose that

book? (People enjoy talking about their favorite books, and by their choice you can learn a lot about them.)

3) I'm doing an informal survey. What do you (or you folks) think is the most important event (or invention) of the twentieth century? (People love to think about such challenging questions.)

A final mingle method worth mentioning is to be your honest, vulnerable self. You can walk up to a person at a party and simply say, "I don't know many people here and you looked like a friendly person I'd like to meet. Hi, my name is Jonathan" (put out your hand to shake). If you want, you can then proceed to ask him or her a question. People react very positively to such a straightforward approach. But whatever mingle method you use, you'll be amply rewarded. It simply feels good to connect with people. After all, connecting with people is what love and good business is all about.

27: Get the Opposite Sex to Value You

The Man/Woman Distinction

B ooks such as John Gray's *Men are From Mars, Women Are From Venus* have popularized the notion that men and women are very different. Yet, from my experience as a counselor, I see that men and women still don't get it. For the most part, we still think that the opposite sex is, or should be, just like us. It ain't gonna happen. Men and women are different because of a million years of evolution. They have different needs, desires, and hopes. Just because modern-day society gives men and women similar opportunities does not mean they have become alike. The more you know why and how men and women are different, the more you can use this information to have successful relationships.

Before exploring how men and women are different, it's useful to know *why* they have unique needs and desires. Understanding why someone is different than you can help alleviate the annoyance that can come from distinct world views. I had this lesson clarified to me recently as I walked my dog down the street near my house. Without any warning, someone walked into me from behind. Well, I was quite annoyed until I turned around to see who it was. It was a blind man with a cane. Since I now understood how such a thing could happen, my annoyance immediately disappeared. Likewise, my hope is that as you understand why the opposite sex behaves differently than you, you'll be more accepting of how they act.

Let's begin with men. For the last million years (except the last relatively few), men have been the hunters and protectors. It was a man's job to risk his life for his tribe by trying to kill animals for food. If a man was unsuccessful at that, he would often be ostracized from the tribe and sometimes starve to death. If a man was successful, he was considered the hero to the entire tribe, and was given special privileges. For example, "successful" men, those who were the meanest and best at killing animals and/or warring tribesmen, got to have sex with whatever women they wanted. In this way, the most aggressive, least "sensitive" men got to pass down their genes to the next generation.

How can this perspective help us nowadays? To begin with, it can help clarify why men have a hard time being emotionally vulnerable and sensitive. Caring, sensitive men weren't so good at killing, and therefore got less opportunities to mate and pass down their genes. In addition, this explains why "success" is so important to men. In the past, only the successful men got to eat well or mate. When someone nags at a man or tells him he's a failure in some manner, unknowingly he or she is giving him a message that, on a subconscious level, threatens his survival. That's why men can rarely admit they are wrong. Their whole underlying psychology is to avoid mistakes and become the hero. When women (or other men) build up a man's ego rather than try to tear it down, he's more energized. After all, historically men would even risk their lives to become a hero.

The evolution of women has been completely different than that of men. Historically, a woman's job was to take care of her kids while the father searched for food. Her survival, and the survival of her kids depended on having a man who was willing to stick by her side. In order to get a successful man to stay with her, a woman's best bet was to look beautiful. If a woman was pretty enough, she was practically assured of having several brutish men willing to risk their lives for her. If a woman was average looking, or not special in some other way, men were more likely to leave them or have sex with other women. This greatly lessened her chances of passing down her own genes. Therefore, women became obsessed with looking beautiful and being special to the men they could attract. Without that "special" bond, they subconsciously knew that their whole survival was at stake.

Once again, it's important to turn this theoretical discussion into practical information. Men need to realize that women need to feel beautiful and special to their mates. When men spend all their time working, or look at other women in a lustful way, it is a direct blow to a women's historical method of survival. That's why women need to be told how beautiful, appreciated, and unique they are. That's why most women like flowers—it's a sign that someone considers them "special." Another way women can be made to feel special is by acknowledging their feelings. In the past, women became experts in the art of nurturing and in being sensitive to feelings, partly due to their job of raising kids. Nowadays, when a man fails to listen to a woman's feelings, she takes it as a sign that he doesn't really care about her. On a deep subconscious level, she may think that her survival is at stake if her man no longer cares about her more than others.

Of course, these statements are gross generalizations about men and women. Yet, there is a lot of evidence to indicate how true they are. For example, the bestselling magazines for women in America are *Better Homes and Gardens* and *Family Circle*. On the other hand, the best selling magazines for men in America are *Playboy* and *Penthouse*. By recognizing and understanding the differences between the sexes, you can get along better with all the people around you. A shorthand way to make use of this information is to ask yourself different questions when trying to get along well with a man or a woman. Since all men want to be a hero, ask yourself, "What can I do to show this man how successful he's already being, and how I appreciate all that he does for me?" As you express this information, men will rise to the occasion because you're giving them what they're hungry for.

To give women what they hunger for, you need to ask a slightly different question. I suggest you ask, "What do I find attractive or beautiful about this woman, and how might I be able to show her how special she is to me?" As you express and act on the insights you get from asking that question, you'll find that women really respond.

These methods and points of view are not meant to be used in a manipulative manner. Instead, the idea is to know what people really want so you can support them in ways they *most* appreciate. When you give the people around you what they truly value, they will be more than happy to give you what you really need and want.

28: Repair Broken Trust

The Science of Creating Safety

Trust is the foundation of any relationship. Whether in a business or intimate relationship, without trust, the whole structure of a personal connection simply falls apart. Even if you communicate with great skill but trust has been broken, you won't get anywhere. The person you're speaking with will simply see your attempts as insincere, and not hear anything you say until trust has been repaired. In my counseling practice, I often see couples who have been hurt so many times by each other that all trust has been destroyed. Teaching them how to communicate better is a necessity, but not quite enough to repair the damage. Additional skills are needed in order to repair trust once it has been broken.

Before discussing how to repair trust, it's useful to understand how it gets broken in the first place. There are two primary ways to damage or destroy the trust in a relationship. First, you can break an agreement with a person. If the agreement is important enough, it may take only one broken promise to destroy the trust you've built together. For example, when one partner has an extramarital affair, it can often leave a relationship in shatters. The second way to damage trust is through hurting a person in various ways. As with broken promises, sometimes a single hurt can decimate trust, such as when a boss verbally abuses an employee. Yet, more commonly there's a pile of little hurts that finally breaks the camel's back. Whatever way trust has been broken, there is a specific process you can go through in order to repair the damage.

Repairing Trust

Think back to a time when someone broke an agreement with you, and you both knew it was his fault. What did you want from him? If you're like most people, you didn't want to hear his excuses and rationalizations. As his excuses babbled out, you probably became even more upset. Instead of giving you excuses, you probably wanted him to acknowledge how hurt or angry you felt, and to take responsibility for being at fault. If a person is upset, it's a good idea to acknowledge their pain, even if you don't know why they're feeling bad. Avoid defending yourself, trying to immediately fix the situation, or turning away. Simply allow this person to feel his or her feelings. Such actions can go a long way in healing the hurt.

To acknowledge someone's hurt or angry feelings, you can ask him or her why they feel bad, and then compassionately listen. Since they're upset, they're likely to vent their feelings in an angry manner. Instead of defending yourself, your job is to see if you can gain a better understanding of what's going on. If there is anything about their story you don't understand, ask them to explain their feelings or story more fully. The more you understand what's going on, the easier it will be to mend the broken trust.

If after listening to someone you still don't understand why they got so upset, you need to further explore their reasoning and feelings. If you have not done something obviously wrong, and yet a person is quite upset, he must have interpreted some behavior or event differently than you. I have found the question, "Why do you think I did (or said) that?" to be profoundly useful in clearing up misunderstandings and hurts. We naturally assume people react to words and behaviors the same way we do, but that's clearly not the case. Only when we know what's really going on in a person's head can we mend the hurts that pile up from misunderstandings. The more information we have, and the more accurate it is, the easier it is to repair the damage.

Once you know why someone is hurt, if it's due to a misunderstanding you can say, "What I meant to say was… (and then say things in a different way.) It's especially useful to say your positive reason or motivation for your actions, such as "I was trying to save you from being hurt" or "I was trying to avoid a problem." By clarifying your intention, the hurt can often be repaired before it hemorrhages into broken trust. If a person's upset isn't due to a misunderstanding, but rather due to a broken agreement, you need to take responsibility for what you did and apologize. This is not an easy thing to do, but because it's so rare, a sincere apology can go a long way toward repairing broken trust.

Once misunderstandings have been cleared up, or appropriate apologies have been given, the last step is to let the person you've hurt know how much you care. When people feel hurt, what hurts is the thought they are being rejected in some way. The obvious antidote to the hurt is telling someone why your relationship is so important to you. As soon as someone is convinced that you really care, trust will be restored. For little misunderstandings, or small errors, it doesn't take long to repair broken trust. But if problems have gone unrepaired for a long time, it can be quite a task to convince someone that you really care. That's why it's always best to heal broken trust as soon as it has been broken.

Sometimes I encounter couples who have recently suffered a big breach of trust, such as an affair, or have piled up so many hurts that only a major act of forgiveness will allow the relationship to move forward. When a partner has been very badly hurt, he will usually need to fully express his hurt and anger before he can really forgive his partner. This is often best done within the context of individual therapy. If the hurt partner tries to directly express her anger and hurt to her mate, it will frequently just turn into an argument. In individual therapy you can get all those bad feelings out without doing additional harm.

Trust, like love, can't be smelled, touched, or tasted, and yet it has massive power. Although it is invisible to our eyes, it is evident in our hearts. You can't have successful relationships without trust. It is important to make consistent efforts to keep the trust between you and others growing strong. The moment you notice trust has been damaged in a relationship, work to repair it as soon as possible. Like a recent wound, broken trust can get infected and spread if the right aid is not quickly applied. Yet, just as bones can grow stronger as they heal from being broken, so can trust grow stronger from being properly repaired.

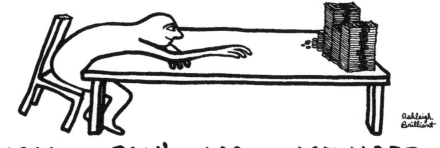

Succeeding at Finances

The financial section of this book is the final section for a reason. Although Western culture values the acquisition of money very highly, money does not make people happy. What makes people happy is a balanced, meaningful life filled with good relationships. When properly used, however, money can be helpful in creating a life filled with health, intimacy, and a passionate sense of purpose. In the chapters that follow, you'll learn many ways to make more money in less time. You'll also learn how to use the money you make to create the life you truly desire, rather than a life simply filled with material distractions and clutter.

In my book, *Real Wealth: A Spiritual Approach to Money and Work,* I talk about how succeeding at finances requires more than just making a lot of money. It also requires finding work you enjoy, having clear goals about how to use money to improve your life, and a sense of how you can become a better human being through achieving your financial goals. In general, people in Western culture have one of two different points of view about money. The first belief is that money is all-important. The second belief is that money isn't important at all. Somewhere between these two extremes lies the truth. Some people need to become less focused on finances, and more focused on creating a meaningful and fulfilling life. Other people need to get *more* focused on finances if they're ever going to create the life they truly desire. Whatever your current financial situation is, you'll find many wonderful shortcuts in the chapters ahead for succeeding in the areas of work and money.

29: Generate Additional Income

The Money-Making Questions

Whether you're looking for a new job that's more profitable and meaningful, or simply want to make additional income at your current job, tapping into your creative potential is a great place to start. Most people think they need to get more degrees or training to make additional income. Nonsense! Perhaps that used to be true, but nowadays, innovation, persistence, problem solving, and marketing ability are often more important than technical training. The good news is that you already possess the resources to tap into each of these four keys for increasing your income. The bad news is that most people don't know how to easily access the resources that lie within them. I have found that asking certain questions can dramatically help people tap into their latent money-making abilities. Once you know these questions, and how to use them properly, you'll find it's easier than ever to create additional income.

Many years ago, I was living in a 1967 Dodge van and making about $4000 a year at odd jobs. One day, I finally reached the point where I was sick and tired of not having any money. To break out of my self-imposed monetary prison, I asked myself a key question: "If my life depended on making a lot more money, what would I do?" Once I got quiet inside and listened to the "still, small voice" within, the answers became obvious. To begin with, I would stop complaining and I'd start learning more about the keys to making money. Therefore, I went to the library and read up on the subject. Next, if my life depended upon having more money, I would overcome my doubts about myself and get a better job or begin my own business. Various other answers came to me, and I began acting on them. Soon, I was doing things which I had never considered before, simply because I was now asking a different question. Within a year, I had made over $40,000.

The issue of money brings up a lot of fear and anxiety for people. When we feel fear, we often lose touch with our ability to solve problems effectively. Therefore, I have found it helpful to ask myself another simple question whenever I feel overwhelmed by a work project or financial situation. The question is, "How can I break this problem down into a bunch of smaller steps?" Soon after moving out of my Dodge van, I decided to do a video on how to have a successful intimate relationship. The problem was I knew nothing about videos, marketing, raising money, or running a business. My girlfriend at the time even chipped in that I knew nothing about having an intimate relationship! There were surely many problems to overcome, and at first I felt overwhelmed. I asked myself, "How can I break this problem down into a bunch of smaller steps?" I soon listed over seventy different small steps I could take toward the completion of the video. As I did each little step, I began to feel confident. To make a long story short, the video became a huge success and launched my career as an author.

To succeed in today's business climate, constant innovation is needed. If you can help your company innovate one of their products or services, you will quickly rise to the top of your field. If you own your own business, your ability to create new, better ways of doing things to serve your customers is your key to prosperity. Yet you may think that thinking in creative ways is beyond your reach. Not true. Creativity and innovation are within your reach if you consistently ask the right question for a long enough period of time. Here's my favorite question to help with this process: "What's a creative new way this job (or service) could potentially be done?" That's it. Asking this question with enough desire and sincerity, along with coming up with a list of several answers, will yield profitable results.

A couple of years ago, I realized that my friends and I rarely had time to read anymore. Since I make a large part of my living by writing books, this realization was a bit depressing. Fortunately, when one door begins to close, it's possible to tune into another one opening— if you know the right question to ask. Therefore, I asked, "What's a creative new way I might write a book that wouldn't take so long to read?" The answer to that question is in your hands right now. I surmised that if I could write books with very brief chapters filled with immediately useful information, people would be able to find the time to read. Of course, this idea only came after I had come up with several other (bad) answers to that same question. When attempting to find new, better ways to handle a situation, coming up with several answers is important. Often, it's only after going through a bunch of poor ideas that gold is struck.

Finally, in order to succeed in business, the ability to market yourself, your product, or your service is key. People are bombarded with so many advertisements nowadays that only the most ingenious marketing strategies are likely to be successful. To help you tap into such ideas, try asking yourself the question, "What would be a new, creative way to convince people of the value of my product or service?" Once again, coming up with a full list of answers is better than just coming up with one or two ideas. Even if your first ideas are truly ridiculous, write them down. Sometimes a very bad idea can be the springboard that triggers a really valuable idea later on.

A couple of years ago, I decided I wanted to do more professional speaking. Although people tell me that speaking is what I do best, it's a very competitive field, and I knew I would have to try some creative marketing ideas. When I asked myself, "What would be a creative way to convince people they should hire me to speak to their company?", I came up with ten suggestions. One of my ideas was to tell them that my regular speaking fee would be reduced by 33 percent if I did not receive a standing ovation at the end of the talk. Since I almost always get a standing ovation at the end of my talks, this bold proposal required nothing new from me. However, it was quite an eye-catcher to the people who read about me and were looking for a speaker. Based on just this one answer to the question I asked, I have already made tens of thousands of extra dollars. Asking the right question can be a richly rewarding use of your time. Whenever you feel stuck in your money-making endeavors, or feel like you're ready to proceed to the next level of prosperity, try asking yourself the four questions below:

1. If my life depended on making a lot more money, what would I do?

2. How can I break this problem down into a bunch of smaller steps?

3. What is a creative, new way this product or service could potentially be done?

4. What would be a creative, new way to convince people of the value of my product or service?

Although asking these questions is deceptively simple to do, the answers you receive, coupled with consistent action, can lead to a whole new level of results and prosperity.

30: Transforming Your Fears Into Money

The Value of Rejection Rewards

In almost any line of work, people find there is something they procrastinate or put off because it makes them uncomfortable or afraid. For example, I often hear that people in various sales occupations avoid making the necessary calls or contacts that will lead to more customers. Usually, the problem is a fear of rejection and/or a fear of failure. Since these fears are the bottleneck blocking so many helpful actions, it's important to explore how to over-come them. Even one thing that you avoid at work due to fear can cost you a promotion, a greatly increased income, or even your job.

One way to overcome your fears is to first realize how much they are currently influenc-ing you. To do this, I find one simple question to be very useful. The question is, "If I had no fear of failure or rejection, and I knew I could not fail, how would I behave differently at work?" Think about it. What specific actions would you do differently? Would you ask for a raise? Would you call upon more clients and ask for more referrals? Would you quit your job and start your own business? Upon contemplating this question, most people begin to real-ize what a major impediment fear can be to their income.

Once you're aware of how you might be different if you had no more fear of failure or rejection, the next step is to create a plan for overcoming these blocks to your prosperity. People refrain from asking for a raise or doing cold calls because they want to avoid the potential pain of facing rejection. To overcome this deeply ingrained tendency, I created a method that moti-vates people to consistently face their fears. I call the method Rejection Rewards, or R.R. for short, because it consists of giving yourself a reward for each and every rejection you receive.

I first came upon this idea when I wanted to get my first book published. I had read that first-time authors have only a one in 1,000 chance of getting their book into print. The thought of a constant stream of rejection letters paralyzed my efforts to move forward. Finally, to overcome my fears, I decided I would treat myself to a professional massage once I had received my first rejection. Once I made that deal with myself, it was only a matter of hours until my first proposal was in the mail. Several weeks later when the rejection came, I had mixed feelings. I was a bit disappointed they didn't want my manuscript, but I was simultaneously delighted that I was to receive a much-needed massage!

In order to stay motivated in the face of constant rejection, I kept giving myself rewards for each manuscript I sent out. I've learned that the greatest resistance to new behavior is at the beginning. For example, in order to get the space shuttle into orbit, it takes 80 percent of its fuel to get it five miles into the air, and only 20 percent of its fuel to get it the other 250 miles into orbit. Therefore, when trying to overcome your fears of failure or rejection, it's important to give yourself a large reward for your first effort. After each effort, you can reduce the size of the reward. By the time I received the tenth rejection on my manuscript, I was rewarding myself with watching a movie on television. The fifteenth publisher I sent my book to was the one that finally said "yes." Of course, since that wasn't a rejection, I had to sacrifice my "reward." Fortunately, by that time I was rewarding myself with a simple candy bar.

As can be seen in the previous example, it is often dogged persistence that pays off. By rewarding yourself for each failure or rejection, it's easier to avoid despair, hopelessness, and burnout. When I coach business clients, I often ask them to figure out how many calls or contacts they typically need to make before they make a sale. One realtor I worked with, Dave, figured he had to talk to forty people by phone or in person for each new listing he received. The task seemed overwhelming until he realized that his commission on each sale (approximately $15,000), divided by each person he had to contact to make that sale (forty people), equaled $375 per person! That was a lot of money to make for only a few minutes of contact. Armed with this new information, Dave began rewarding himself for every fifth contact he made, knowing in the long run that five contacts were worth $1,875. As he treated himself to nice dinners and gadgets for every fifth potential client he talked to, Dave became more motivated to make the cold calls he used to avoid.

Rejection Rewards can make a huge difference in your behavior and income. In Dave's case, instead of begrudgingly making forty calls every other month, he began making forty contacts every other week. Not surprisingly, his income went up by a factor of four, from $60,000 a year, to over $240,000 in a single year!

To make use of this method, simply decide what you tend to avoid at work, and what specific reward(s) you'll give yourself whenever you do something difficult. As in Dave's case, you may reward yourself for filling a certain quota of calls, or as in my case, give yourself a reward for each and every effort you make. Rewards can be anything you enjoy, from a walk in nature to a cruise vacation. It's best to write down the specific deal you're making with yourself so you know exactly when you deserve to indulge. One of the best things about Rejection Rewards is that they diabolically change your attitude about "failure." Instead of leading to paralysis, you learn to accept and even enjoy facing fear as part of the process of success. After all, every step along the way you get to enjoy some kind of reward!

3 I : Sell Your Products Like Wildfire

The Art of Service and Creating Trust

Although the U.S. economy is holding its own, most businesses are noticing that competition keeps heating up. Customers want more service and value for less money. Employers want more done in less time. In this age of frequent downsizing, constant sales, and low profit margins, how can you thrive without sacrificing too much? The answer is to differentiate yourself through establishing superior service. Because people have a lack of time, and they crave genuine human contact, trust and superior service are hidden assets that can go a long way to improving any company's bottom line. In addition, when you or your company become focused on providing customers great service, it makes work more fun. There are few things more rewarding than seeing a customer who is grateful, surprised, and satisfied.

We've all experienced companies who are committed to great service, from Nordstrom's department store to the corner deli. What do these places have in common? I believe there are four ingredients of creating trust and superior service in a business. As you or your company make use of these four keys, you'll find that your customers or clients will be very happy. Satisfied customers keep coming back, and often bring their friends as well. Even if you charge more than your competition, you'll find that service is such a rare commodity nowadays that your clients will be glad to pay a little extra. Everyone wins!

The first key to tapping into your hidden assets is to create a fantastic guarantee for your customers. Several years ago I decided to make a bold statement at one of my workshops.

Speaking from my heart, I told the audience that I truly felt my audio and video tapes could positively impact their life. Then, I went on to state that if they bought any of my products, and they felt the information wasn't worth at least twice what they paid for it, they could send it back to me for a full refund. I went on to say that the refund was good for ten years, and I would even pay the taxes and postage. Well, I literally doubled my sales overnight, and in the last five years, only two books and two tapes have been returned.

How might you create a guarantee that is stated so strongly that it gets the attention of your customers? Anytime you take away the risk to the purchaser, you increase the likelihood of making a sale. Be willing to make your guarantee a little outlandish. After all, if you have a good product or service, it won't be a problem. If people aren't happy with what you sell, then you shouldn't be selling it. I tell my customers that they can even write in my book, try out the methods for years, and if they finally decide it wasn't worth it to them, they can *still* send it back for a full refund. This guarantee pushes them over the edge to a buying decision. My customers get valuable information, and I make more sales. Win, win.

A second ingredient of creating great service is to hire employees committed to giving their best. Some people are just naturals at helping people, while others are not. When people give their best, it simply feels better than doing things in a rushed and sloppy manner. Therefore, it's important that employees be encouraged and rewarded for service and impeccability, instead of just efficiency. Rewards tend to give you more of what you want, so if you can figure out some way to reward your employees (or yourself) for treating people superbly, you'll do well in the long run.

Next, if you want to establish a bond of trust with your customers, you need to be able to admit your mistakes, make a clear apology, and then commit yourself to doing the job right. Not long ago, I went to a printer who managed to foul up a printing job I had given him. Upon seeing my slightly tarnished letterhead, an employee tried to blame my graphics person for the mistake. Fortunately, the owner of the shop overheard and stepped in. He looked at the letterhead, apologized for the sloppy work, and said he'd do it again right away. I was impressed. He now had a customer who was loyal. Having successfully resolved a potential conflict with him, I now felt that I could trust him in the future.

A final key that can help create a sense of superior service is to do something extra to surprise your client or customer. I do this all the time simply because it makes me feel good. As an added bonus, I've noticed it has a tremendous positive impact on people. For example, when I see patients in my psychotherapy practice, at the end of the session I'll often give them a free book or tape. It doesn't cost me much, but it's so unexpected that it has quite an impact on their relationship with me. I also tell them they can call me anytime on the phone for free if they're having a particularly rough time. In twelve years of private practice, I've only received three such calls, yet several patients have told me that this sincere offer "sold" them on having me as their therapist.

A few years ago, a friend of mine insisted I go to Nordstrom's to buy some new clothes. Despite my fears of how expensive I thought Nordstrom's was, I finally went. It was my first joyous shopping experience. While waiting to see some clothes specially selected for me, I was offered some fresh-squeezed orange juice by a salesperson. The pianist at a nearby piano (in the store) asked me if I had a favorite piece of music I would like to hear. While sipping on orange juice and listening to Bach's *Ode to Joy,* I thought to myself, "This is what shopping should be!" Although such things don't happen every time I go to Nordstrom's, the fact that I'm sometimes surprised keeps me coming back. Gambling casinos also know that occasional pleasant surprises get people coming back for more. The same could be true in your business.

The four keys I've listed— offering a great guarantee, giving your best, admitting and correcting your mistakes, and pleasantly surprising your customer (or boss) will infuse your work with a higher sense of meaning and purpose. As these keys create more trust and service with those that you work for, your bottom line and your attitude will both prosper.

32: Double Your Income in Three Years

The Coaching Team Commitment

If you're serious about making more money, then you're going to need help. Setting clear, achievable goals is a good start. Having a burning desire will also help, as will talent and good technical and social skills. Yet, the two biggest factors in helping you to quickly double your income will be the ability to act consistently and the skill of seeking assistance from other people. As author Tony Robbins has said, "A lot of people know what to do, but few people do what they know." An effective way to make sure you take persistent action and receive help from others is by creating a Coaching Team. A Coaching Team is a group of two to eight people who are committed to achieving their goals at an accelerated rate. By following the simple guidelines set out here for forming your own team, you should be able to double your income in three years or less. Of course, if you have goals other than making more money, you'll find that they can also be achieved more quickly through this method.

The basic structure of the Coaching Team is simple. Once a month, the entire team gets together to choose new partners, help each other out with new ideas, and talk about how it's going. Each week, every person on the team agrees to talk to their coaching partner for that month (in person or on the phone) for at least ten minutes. During this time, you help each other to set realistic goals for the upcoming week, review how things went during the previous week, and even "coach" each other in how to better handle the challenges you each face. Good questions to ask during these coaching sessions include the following:

1. How did you do with the goals and commitments you made last week?

2. What are the current goals you're working on, and how might you be able to move forward with them during the upcoming week?

3. Is there any area in your life that you feel stuck? If so, what do you see as the problem? (Feel free to offer advice or new perspectives.)

4. Are there some things you can schedule into your upcoming week to help you achieve your goals, especially things you might normally procrastinate on or avoid?

5. What are you willing to commit to do this week no matter what?

I have found that when people know they are going to be accountable to someone else at the end of each week, their level of productivity skyrockets. Besides the motivating factor of being accountable to someone else, the weekly talk with your coaching partner can lead to valuable inspiration and insights. During your coaching conversations, you should feel free to offer advice or other questions when talking with your partner. When people face challenges, they often get locked into "tunnel vision" and lose the ability to think creatively about how to overcome their problems. Your additional questions, encouragement, and perspective will frequently be the key ingredient to help your partner move forward. As soon as you're done coaching your partner, they can proceed to help you in a similar manner. Usually, the entire conversation takes about fifteen minutes.

The goals you work on during these coaching conversations need not have to do with your career or finances, nor do you and your partner need similar goals. I was "partners" with one man for over a year. He was interested in increasing his income by 40 percent in a year (which he did), and I was focused on improving my health and deepening my level of peace. Although we weren't close friends and we had different goals, we really supported each other. I remember how good it felt to coach someone and see them make continued progress.

Coaching has proven so effective that there are now professional "personal coaches" who are hired to help people achieve their goals. Of course, it can be expensive to hire a personal coach. I think the simple act of finding a friend, mate, or coworker and asking him or her on a weekly basis the previous five questions is usually sufficient.

Besides the weekly coaching conversations, I suggest you get together with your partner and the other team members once every month for a group meeting. During this time, you can briefly mention how it's going, and ask for help from your other teammates regarding your goals. When I've been in such groups, we've normally given each person about fifteen minutes to ask for help with any problem or situation in their life. Then, everyone throws out as many ideas and suggestions as they can think of to help the person whose turn it is to receive. I know that when I've faced problems in my life, I often fail to see obvious or creative solutions to my situation. Yet by receiving help from friends I know and trust, I've often been able to benefit from their ideas and wisdom. Just one good idea from someone on your coaching team can make a world of difference. In addition, I enjoy the feeling of helping other people achieve their goals.

To get the most out of a coaching team group or a coaching partner, it's important to clearly define the areas you would like help with. Completing the sentence, "The problem I would like help with is..." is a good way to begin. It can also be useful to briefly explain what you've already tried, and any relevant history that may help others tailor their answers to your specific situation. Two heads are indeed better than one, and several heads working together can often overcome difficult situations with ease. When among several people in a coaching group, it's a good idea to set a timer for fifteen or twenty minutes per person so that everyone will have an equal length of time to receive feedback.

Many of the most successful men and women in history have made use of weekly accountability sessions and coaching groups as a way to accelerate their progress toward important goals. In this day and age of rapid change, learning how to make use of other people's support is more critical than ever. Besides achieving your goals rapidly, deep friendships can develop in such supportive environments. It feels good to get and receive help. Once you give it a try, I think you'll recognize its profound value. Allow friends or coworkers who might be interested in this process to read this chapter. If they like the idea, agree to have weekly coaching conversations for a month to see how it goes. If it goes well, keep it going. You'll be amazed at the results you get.

33: Retire at a Young Age

The Secrets of Saving Money

North Americans are not known for saving money. Unlike Japanese or Europeans, we consistently spend more than we make. This is a problem—spending more than you make is the first rule of bankruptcy, not retirement. If you want to retire at a young age (or retire comfortably at an old age), it helps to know how most people have done it and then copy their strategy. From studying various people who have stopped working for money by the time they were forty-five, I've seen that almost all of them have done five things similarly. My hope is that as you do these behaviors, you'll be able to get similar results.

Many people assume that the way to retire early is to make a lot of money at a high-stress job. This does not seem to be the case. People who go this route usually find themselves caught up in a fast-paced lifestyle and spend all the money they make. A better way to save a lot of money is to simply spend less than you make, even if you don't make very much. Experts in the field of finances often suggest taking 10 percent of all you earn and investing it. Even a person who worked their whole life at *minimum wage,* but consistently invested 10 percent of their salary in the stock market, would have a net worth of over a million dollars at age sixty-five. Of course, since virtually no one stays at minimum wage, investing 10 percent of your earnings can get you to a million dollars way before you become a senior citizen.

Since investing 10 percent of your earnings is a formula that works so well in creating an early retirement, there are only two more things you need to do to retire early. First, you need to learn some practical ways to help you save 10 percent of your earnings. And second, you need to know how to invest that money wisely so that it will create a maximum return for you later on. Let's begin by looking at how you can save 10 percent of what you make.

No matter what your income level, you can save 10 percent of what you make. I know it doesn't seem possible, but it is. How? I know of four very simple money-saving ideas that will help you save and invest the "extra" 10 percent:

1) Put a "waiting period" on nonessential purchases. If you see something you want to buy

(other than food or other essentials), simply hold off buying it for two weeks. If after two weeks you still feel like you want or need it, then buy it. Many of our purchases are bought on impulse and are not really needed. This method will help you to avoid impulse buying. You'll be amazed at how much less junk you bring home by simply creating a "waiting period."

2) Never buy luxury items with a credit card and learn to avoid all credit card debt. If you have to pay interest on a credit card, you'll never get ahead financially. Credit cards take the "sting" out of purchases. However, you want to face and feel the "sting" of any major purchase. After all, each unnecessary purchase further delays your dream of financial independence. When you pay cash for items, you'll be more conservative in what you buy.

3) Understand why you want to buy something. Basically, we buy nonessential items because we think they will help us to feel a certain way. People buy a sports car for the feeling of adventure. People buy fancy clothes to help them feel confident or sexy. Unfortunately, many of the feelings we try to get via material goods can more easily be experienced through other means. For example, an expensive sports car can help you to feel excited and fully alive, but so can a good movie at a small fraction of the cost. An expensive vacation can help you feel relaxed, but so can a massage or an hour of meditation. Therefore, before making big purchases, it's helpful to ask yourself, "What might be a less expensive way I can feel the same feelings that this purchase would give me?" If something occurs to you, try it out. It may save you a lot of money.

4) Do as much as you can on barter. (See chapter 6 for more about barter). For almost all of humanity's history, bartering goods, information, and services has been how things got done. Despite our current money-based economy, bartering is still a great way to get things done. In addition, it's tax-free, helps create friendships, saves time, and can be a great way to save money. Instead of paying for your next income tax preparer, car repair, or house painting, see if you can find someone who would exchange their skills for some of yours.

Besides saving 10 percent of what you earn and investing it, a person desiring early retirement needs to invest their money intelligently. How to wisely invest your money depends on factors such as your age, where you live, the economy, your marital status, and other factors. Yet, over the long term, two investments in particular have almost always out performed other strategies. They are owning your own house and investing in the stock market. Owning your own house is useful because it greatly reduces your taxes, is a forced way to save (your mortgage builds equity), and the price of houses almost always goes up over the long term. If you're not currently a homeowner, studying how and where to buy your own house is a good investment of your time.

Secondly, over long periods of time, the stock market has traditionally provided higher returns than other forms of investments. Money market accounts, savings in banks, and other forms of investment tend to barely outpace inflation, whereas the stock market has done much better than inflation over the long term. Since every year leads to unique market and economic conditions, your best weapon is information. There are plenty of good books about investing, such as Charles Givens *Creating Wealth.* You will receive a very high return on a small investment of time if you familiarize yourself with typical investment strategies. The skills presented here can potentially help you to save and invest thousands of extra dollars per year. After you retire at an early age, while you're sipping a martini on the beach, remember to thank me.

34: Achieve Both Wealth and Peace

Inner and Outer Goals

Setting and achieving goals is perhaps the most documented technique for manifesting what you want, efficiently and effectively. Since writing your goals is so powerful, it's important to know precisely what you want to create so you will be pleased when you get it. If you don't specify your dreams clearly enough, you can end up creating a nightmare. Sometimes people who write down their goals *do* create a life that is out of harmony. Why? Because their goals are all outward goals, such as making more money. Yet manifesting more money is of little good if it's created at the cost of your time, relationships, and peace of mind. Therefore, I think it's best to create what I call "balanced goals." *Balanced goals are goals that have both an internal and an external element to them.* For example, if you want more money, it can be helpful to know *why* you want it. If you realize it's to have more peace of mind, then why not make it a goal to create more peace of mind in your life *while* you make more money?

There are many advantages to creating balanced goals. First of all, by knowing both the internal and external target you're aiming for, it's more likely you'll hit the bull's-eye. Some people who go only for the external target, such as making money, end up completely missing the internal target. They make millions but they don't get what they really wanted, such as more peace of mind. Another advantage of balanced goals is the fact that they help people experience what they really want more quickly. After all, people really *do* want more peace, and having more money is just *one* method of creating it. By exploring more ways to create inner peace, a person is almost certain to have greater success. A third advantage of balanced goals is that they help people to grow spiritually and financially at the same time. Creating balanced goals is a way to produce balance within ourselves so we can better create harmony in our lives.

Several years ago, I had a wealthy client named Steven who came to me for counseling. His stated goal was that he wanted to make more money. After asking him a few questions, I found out that he made over $200,000 a year! When I asked him why he wanted more money, he said, "If I just had more money I could finally get the respect and feeling of success I've always wanted." From my perspective, he didn't need more money, he needed a greater sense of self-esteem. Yet had I told him he needed to work on the internal goal of increased self-esteem, he probably would have walked out of my office. Instead, I suggested we create a balanced goal. We authored a plan to raise his income and a separate plan for raising his self-esteem. The synergy of our two plans working together created amazingly quick results. As he worked on his self-esteem, he made more money, and as he made more money, it further elevated his self-esteem. Two goals working in synchrony are much better than one goal alone.

To create a balanced goal, you need to know two things. First, you need to know exactly what you'd like to manifest in the material world. Second, you want to identify what you hope to experience as a result of achieving your external goal. In my interactions with Steven, his desired outer goal was more money, but his desired inner goal was a feeling of respect and success. The easiest way to know what inner goal is appropriate for you is to ask yourself the following question: "What feeling do I hope to experience as a result of achieving my external goal (such as more money, a house, etc.)?" Once you know what feeling or experience you ultimately want to have, make having more of that experience the focus of your inner goal. What follows is an example of how you might go through the four-step process for achieving an inner goal. To better illustrate this process, I'll use my interaction with a client named Sarah as an example:

1) Write down your inner goal. To know your inner goal, ask yourself: "What feeling do I hope to experience as a result of achieving my external goal?" When I asked Sarah this question, she eventually realized she wanted more comfort and security.

2) Write down the criteria that the goal has been adequately achieved. In the case of inner goals, I suggest people create an "intuitive scale" to measure how they're doing. Ask yourself,

"On a 1 to 10 scale (10 representing the best possible), how much of my inner goal (in Sarah's case, how much comfort and security) do I currently have in my life?" When I asked Sarah this question, she said she was "about a 4." Then I asked her, "Where do you want to be on a 1 to 10 scale, and by when?" She responded, "I'd like to be at a level 7 five months from today."

3) Brainstorm steps you could take to help you move toward achieving what you ultimately want. Ask other people how they might go about achieving a similar goal. The more ideas you come up with, the better. You should be able to fill in this sentence: "Six or more things I could do to help me on the path of achieving my goal are . . . ." When I asked Sarah this question, she came up with the following list:

1. Ask people who experience a deep sense of comfort and security in their life what their secret is.

2. Learn to meditate so I can quiet my mind and feel more secure within myself.

3. Listen to hypnosis tapes to quiet my mind and feel less worry.

4. Take a self-defense class so I know I can always defend myself if I have to.

5. Read a book on how to have more confidence and feel more comfortable in social situations.

6. Ask two friends what they think would help me increase the level of comfort and security I feel in my life.

4) Do the activities on your brainstorm list in a logical order until you've achieved the goal—or need to create a new plan.

Notice that in the example with Sarah, I had her create an internal way to measure her progress toward more security and comfort. You can always improve what you can measure. Although creating an "intuitive 1 to 10 scale" is not absolutely precise, I've found that people say it works surprisingly well in measuring their progress. All you need to do is rate, on an internal 1 to 10 scale, how you're currently doing in the area you want to work on. Then, about once a week ask yourself, "How am I now doing (on a 1 to 10 scale)?" Hopefully, you'll see gradual improvement. If not, it may mean you need to do different tasks in order to be more successful.

For the best results, keep your goals on a sheet of paper that you can see every day. About once a week or so, read over your plan and see how you're doing. See if you can schedule any more steps from your plan into the upcoming week.

By taking small actions each week on her internal and external goals, Sarah was able to achieve both her goals. In fact, she achieved her internal goal (creating more comfort and security) much faster than she expected. Sarah reported to me that her newfound comfort with herself assisted her on her job, which eventually led to the increase in pay she desired. When people create balanced goals, they often work in a synergistic manner that leads to extraordinary results. As you set balanced goals, you'll soon notice that your life feels more centered, balanced, and harmonious. With the right method, it *is* possible to experience both wealth *and* peace.

35: Easily Achieve Your Goals

The Twelve Common Goal-Setting Mistakes

Recently, I was listening to a tape series that detailed the lives of dozens of great men and women throughout history. Although the times they each lived in and challenges they faced were different, one theme kept standing out in the stories of their lives: almost all of them had set specific goals for themselves. From Benjamin Franklin to Mother Teresa, creating clear and meaningful goals stood out as the one ingredient that most people who succeed in life have in common.

Since goal-setting is so powerful, why doesn't everyone do it? Because we're lazy and we haven't been told how to do it in an easy and effective manner. Even people who write down their goals often do things that interfere with getting the results they desire. As a seminar leader that teaches goal setting, I've noticed that people tend to make the same twelve errors when pursuing their dreams. To help you avoid these common pitfalls, I have listed each of them, along with a brief explanation as to how to make sure you don't fall into the same trap:

1. Forgetting to write down your goals, and/or not having a clear criteria for their success—including when you would like your goal (or part of the goal) completed by. To avoid this problem, get out a piece of paper as soon as you're done reading this and simply fill in the sentence "A goal I'd like to achieve is _____, and I'd like to achieve it by _____." (provide a specific date).

2. Setting goals that are unrealistic in order to make up for all the time you may have wasted in the past. Unrealistic goals lead to discouragement when they are not met, and this could result in giving up completely. Instead, make sure you feel you can achieve this goal. Even be willing to set a goal that might be overly easy to achieve. You can always build on your successes.

3. Setting too many goals at once in order to make up for being behind, which could lead to discouragement or a lack of focus. Rather than set a lot of goals, why not simply try one or two. If you start making consistent progress toward these, then you can think about making other goals.

4. Failure to ask other people or experts for help in how best to achieve your goal, or using an inefficient or unusable method to manifest what you want. If you're facing East looking for a sunset, you're going to have problems. When people don't ask experts for a good approach to achieve a goal, they often come up with ideas that don't work effectively. Avoid this pitfall by seeking the advice of experts, whether from books or from people you know.

5. Failure to break each goal into small, easily doable steps. When you forget to do this, there is a tendency to become overwhelmed by the size of the task, and eventually to give up. To avoid this error, simply brainstorm a list of every small or big task that might be helpful to achieve your goal. Then take the big tasks and break them into smaller, bite-sized activities.

6. Not having your step-by-step plan written down and in daily sight. Once you have a list of tasks to do, come up with a logical order in which to do them and put them on a single sheet of paper. This will help you feel organized and will visually remind you of what to do next.

7. Not anticipating obstacles, or not being committed enough to overcome them. Obstacles will happen—you can count on it. In fact, writing down the obstacles you anticipate, along with how you plan to get around them when they occur, can help you overcome them.

8. Forgetting to put the next step toward the completion of your goal into your calendar or "to do" list. Whenever you complete one of the steps on your goal sheet, it's time to schedule the *next* task into your daily planner. Even if you can only spend an hour a week, you don't want to lose momentum toward achieving your goal. By writing it down into your "to do" list, you can feel confident that it'll get done.

9. Becoming too impatient to do just a little bit each week toward the completion of your goal, thereby becoming inconsistent in your actions. Manifesting your dreams takes time. More importantly, it takes consistency. If you're willing to take small steps over a long period

of time, you'll be amazed at what you can create. If you try to do too much too quickly, you'll likely just burn out and then give up.

10. Failing to create an effective system to stay motivated and consistent in your actions until your goal is achieved. In order to stay motivated over time, it helps to have someone who can inspire you and help hold you accountable (see chapters 15 and 32 for more on this). By having a buddy you can talk to on a weekly basis regarding your progress, you'll find that you'll be much more likely to stay consistent in your actions.

11. Lack of flexibility when something doesn't work quite right, which can lead to giving up instead of making the appropriate adjustments to your plan. After working on your goals for awhile, you may find that your original plan doesn't work. What then? If you're flexible in your approach to solving problems, you'll simply come up with a new plan.

12. Forgetting to celebrate your achievements, thereby never getting the sense of satisfaction and success that you deserve. Some people don't even realize when they've achieved their goals. It's hard to get motivated to achieve new goals if you've never fully celebrated your accomplishments in the past. Rewarding yourself for a job well done will help you to feel good, and it will also help you be motivated to achieve new goals.

Goal-setting is an amazing technology, but like all technology, you need to know how to handle it properly. (For additional information on goals, see chapter 34). If you find that you have fallen in one of the twelve pitfalls, then take the appropriate action to pull yourself out as fast as possible. Achieving your goals is like being a shark: if you're still for too long, the goal will die. Keep moving forward, building on the momentum of what you've already accomplished. Before you know it, your dreams will be a reality.

36: Tap Into Your Creative Potential

The Art of Innovation

It used to be that creativity was something consigned to mad scientists, artists, and advertising departments. Think again. Nowadays, company profits are largely based on innovations that give them a slight edge over their competition. The ability to come up with creative ideas is one of the most valued commodities an employee can offer his or her company. Innovative thinking, however, is not nurtured in our schools. In fact, it is trained out of us. George Land, a scientist who studied creativity found that 98 percent of five-year-olds ranked as "highly creative," whereas only 12 percent of fifteen-year-olds did. His conclusion was that "noncreative behavior is learned." Fortunately, *creative* behavior can also be learned or, more accurately, relearned.

Buckminster Fuller called the process of innovation "cosmic fishing." I will briefly describe several methods of coming up with creative solutions to problems. Once you know these tools, you'll be amazed at how many new, fun, and effective ideas you can create out of thin air. By the simple act of using these tools to dive deeply within your own mind, you can pull out solutions and ideas that will greatly enrich your professional and personal life.

Before exploring specific creativity-enhancing games, let's look at two simple ideas that can increase your overall I.Q. (Imagination Quotient). First, since much of today's innovation requires a certain amount of technical information, it's important to immerse yourself in the appropriate pool of knowledge. For example, if you want to write a story about horses, it can help to read books and watch videos about horses, as well as go and ride some. As you dive into this sea of experience, some creative ideas are bound to percolate up from the depths of your subconscious mind.

A second concept that can lead to increased innovation and creativity is to become like a child again. After all, they score much higher on creativity tests than adults. What do children do? They take time each day for play, mischief, and breaks to do nothing but have fun. They see things with curiosity and a sense of wonder. They explore. They use props to help fire up their imagination, whether it's talking to their dolls or shooting with their toy guns. To a four-year-old, a spoon isn't just a spoon. It's also a nose scruncher, a food flinger, and a scalp massager. As you let the playful child within you out, you'll find yourself thinking in new ways, and enjoying the sense of freedom that comes from exploring new paths.

There are many games or exercises that can help to stimulate your creative potential. The simple act of clearly defining a problem on paper can serve to focus the mind in creative ways. For instance, let's say you have a goal to get a promotion and pay raise at work. You can state at the top of a piece of paper, "My goal (or my problem) is I want to get a pay raise and promotion at work." Then try to come up with twenty ideas that can help you achieve your goal or solve your problem. The first few solutions should be easy. The next few ideas shouldn't be too bad, but the last five to ten will likely stimulate much creative thought. They don't even have to be good ideas, you just need twenty of them. Often bad ideas lead to good ideas, so write everything down and see what gets stimulated. When done in a group, this simple excerise frequently results in one person coming up with ideas that help stimulate innovation from someone else.

Another technique to help heighten creativity is to ask yourself or a group of people innovation-enhancing questions. For example, once a problem is defined, you might ask, *"What else is the problem?"* You can keep asking this question until you see the problem in a different light. Instead of seeing the problem as not making enough money from your job, perhaps you could see it as spending too much, or failing to make a good return on your investments. How you define a problem can stimulate different creative responses, so it's helpful to define it in varied ways.

Other creativity-enhancing questions include the ones below. By coming up with several answers to each question, you can further stimulate your creative ideas:

1. What would be another way of approaching this situation, goal, or problem?

2. What are the hidden assumptions we're making here, and what if one of those assumptions changed?

3. How might a four-year-old look at this?

4. How might the word _____ relate to this goal or problem?

For question number four, you can simply go to a dictionary and pick out a random noun, such as the word "banana." If your problem were how to make more money, you might come up with ideas such as:

1. I could start bringing fruit or other snacks to work for my coworkers and boss, and thereby get on everyone's good side.

2. I could eat more fruits and vegetables, and thereby have more energy to go to night school and get a better job.

3. I could bring a banana and other food to work each day instead of eating at the expensive diner across the street.

As you can see, there is virtually no end to the ideas that can spring forth from simple questions.

A final tool for helping you think in new and expanded ways is from a book by Edward de Bono called *Six Thinking Hats*. In this book, de Bono suggests that when thinking about a situation, it can help to use six deliberate thinking strategies to gain a wider perspective and stimulate new ideas. His six "hats" or thinking strategies are delineated as follows:

White: facts, figures, and objective information such as a computer could process.

Red: emotions or feelings about a goal or problem; how you feel about the situation.

Green: creative, new ways of looking at a problem; new alternatives and approaches.

Yellow: positive assessments, possible benefits, optimistic thinking.

Black: pessimistic thinking, what could go wrong, possible problems, risks and dangers.

Blue: the director of the thinking process, controller of what hats to put on and when.

In using this method, an individual or a group would put on different "hats" or thinking styles to get a full view of a problem or desired goal. For example, if the problem were to figure out if you should apply for a new job, each thinking style would give you additional information.

While in the white hat you might see that you only have $3,000 in savings, in the red hat you would realize you're afraid to quit your old job, but in the green hat you might realize you could temporarily try a second job, or look for another job while keeping your old one. As you go through each thinking style, you increase the likelihood of stimulating useful ideas you may have missed through your normal thinking process. When done in a group, it's a good idea to give one person the blue hat and have him or her direct when everyone will "put on" one of the other hats. In this way, everyone's thinking style can feed off the other participants, and lead to amazing realizations that could not be achieved alone.

Now that we're beginning the twenty-first century, we need to use our full creative potential in order to keep up in this fast-changing world. The tools described here will help you reach your goals and solve problems more quickly and effectively than you may have ever thought possible. So don't let your creativity stagnate or hibernate and become second-rate. Instead, innovate, elevate, incubate, scintillate, illustrate, and impregnate your thinking till it becomes first-rate.

37: Pay Less Income Tax

The Legal Deduction Game

What is the biggest expense you will have in your entire life? Health care? Children? A house? Nope. Income taxes. At least 25 percent of all the money you ever make will go to the government in the form of various taxes. If you are armed with the right expertise, however, you can avoid unnecessary taxes and enjoy tax loopholes that will profoundly reduce the amount you pay in taxes. So why doesn't everybody use these "loopholes?" Because people are lazy, some of these strategies are a pain in the ass to learn about, and some require discipline to use. To make things easy on you, I'll discuss four of the most effective and common tax reduction strategies. This is not meant to be a thorough analysis of the subject—I recommend two good books later in this chapter. Rather, my aim is to convince you that these ways to reduce your tax bill are worth looking into. If after reading this it inspires you to take action in one of the ways I suggest, I will feel like I've done my duty.

The first way to reduce your tax bill is to buy a house. For years I was adamant about not owning a house. I wanted to be a free spirit, able to come and go as I please. Then someone laid out the numerous financial advantages. I was convinced, and I've never regretted it. In terms of taxes, buying a house makes sense because the interest on the mortgage you pay on your house is tax deductible, whereas your monthly rent is not. If you have a $150,000 mortgage at 7 percent interest, that means your monthly payment is about $1000, most of which is tax deductible. That's over ten grand a year in tax deductions. Hallelujah! In addition, the money you pay on your mortgage builds equity as you slowly pay off the principle, whereas the money you pay in rent disappears into a black hole. If coming up with an initial down payment is a problem, there are numerous books on ways to buy houses for little or no money down. Also, buying a condo can be a bit easier than a house, and yet still has the same tax advantages. It's worth looking into.

Tax reduction strategy number two is Individual Retirement Accounts, better known as IRAs. IRAs are a great tax incentive "gift" the U.S. government offers its citizens in order to entice us into saving money for our retirement. There are two commonly used types of IRAs, regular and Roth. They have many similarities. Both types have a maximum amount you can put into your account of $2,000 per year. Both allow you to take money out starting at age fifty-nine. Both allow you to withdraw cash without owing the 10 percent early withdrawal penalty if you are buying your first home, paying for a college education for you, your spouse, or your child, or paying certain medical expenses. Yet with the regular IRA, the money you put in each year is tax deductible and earns money tax-free until removed, at which time you pay taxes on whatever you have. With the Roth IRA, the money you put in is *not* tax deductible but it earns money tax-free and is also tax-free *when taken out*. If you can afford to put $2,000 (or anything) into an IRA each year, the tax savings that accrue over time are substantial. Check with your local bank or financial planner for more details as to which type of IRA might best apply to you, or you can consult Vanguard's web page to help to figure out which is best for you at: www:vanguard.com.

A third method of reducing your tax bill is to put money into a 401k plan, which is basically a retirement or pension plan in which your employer usually matches the amount you put in. In such a plan, you pay no tax on the amount the employer puts in, the money you put in is deducted from your taxable income, and all the money is tax-free when you take it out, which can be when you're fired, quit, or are age fifty-nine and a half. The amount you can put into a 401k is often based on the particular plan, but whatever you put in reduces your tax bracket. Since various plans have unique rules and regulations, it's best to consult your employer for the details of the plan they offer.

If you're in business for yourself, you can put money into a pension or profit-sharing plan. In this plan, an employer agrees to pay a specific share of profits to all employees. Therefore, this situation is best for someone with no employees (or at least very few), since you have to pay the same percentage to each employee. The advantage of this type of plan is that you can put a lot of money into it and whatever you put in is tax-free. Since there are numerous rules about these plans, it's best to check with your accountant to see if this might be a good match for you.

The last tax-reduction strategy I want to discuss is the advantages of going into business for yourself. Besides the fact that it's hard to become rich when working for others, being in business for yourself allows you to deduct many of the expenses related to having a business. For example, if you have a home office that is exclusively devoted to business, you can deduct the amount you pay on that space. You can even deduct anything directly connected to the business you're in, such as education, workshops, books, business travel, and a portion of your auto expenses. If you're in a business that you love, then you're in the fortunate position of being able to deduct the cost of things such as seminars and computer programs that you would naturally want to buy anyway. Since I do a lot of speaking to corporations and associations across the country, I get to visit a lot of cities and have my travel expenses deducted. Isn't the government good? As always, it's a good idea to check with an accountant to discern exactly what is deductible and what is not when filing your tax statements.

Few people like to get into the nitty-gritty details of pension plans, tax forms, IRA regulations, and all the other minutia of modern-day economics. However, knowing this information and how it can apply to you can save you tens of thousands of dollars over the course of your lifetime. Perhaps it will take you ten hours of research to learn what you need to know about the tax-reduction strategies that would work best for you. If those ten hours of research lead to an extra $100,000 of tax-free money over the course of your life (which is easily possible), then, in effect, you'd be making $10,000 an hour for the time you spend researching!

That's decent pay. So despite the fact that you may hate looking into the benefits and disadvantages of each of the programs I briefly mentioned here, it's probably worth your while. Decide on how you can get more information. You can begin by looking at the updated yearly books, *How to Pay Zero Taxes* by Jeff Schnepper or *Make More Money* by the editors of *Money Magazine.* Uncle Sam is rich enough. Don't give him any more than he's entitled to.

38: Sell Like the Pros

The Art of Integrity Selling

We're all salespeople at some time in our life. When we were kids, we tried to sell our mom or dad on why we should get to stay up late. Now, we sell to our boss, our customers, or to our own kids on why they should not stay up past their bedtime. While we all try to sell something, some people are just a lot more effective at it than others. What are the practical principles and techniques that the pros use to sell? What *really* works when selling, and what is just manipulative gimmicks and hype? I believe there are a few proven fundamentals to selling that can be easily learned. As you use these ideas, you'll notice your kids willingly going to bed on time, as well as your business awakening to new heights.

1) Build rapport with the person to whom you hope to sell. In other chapters in this book I talk about various ways of building rapport (see chapters 23, 25, and 26). At its core, rapport

is the art of getting people to like you and trust you. Before people hear a sales pitch, they want to know if you have their best interests in mind. Although there are several ways to do this, one simple way to get a person to trust you is to simply listen carefully to whatever he or she says. As you acknowledge and empathize with what someone says, they will tend to feel more at ease and safe with you. Statements such as "I can appreciate how you..." or "I understand how that would feel..." help to build trust. At the very least, it shows that you understand what they're saying and can listen to their needs.

2) Understand what motivates people. As I've mentioned in other sections, people do things to avoid pain and/or to gain pleasure. Selling is largely the process of getting people to believe that your product, service, or idea will bring them more pleasure than pain. However, since people are primarily motivated by the desire to avoid pain, it's important to first get people in touch with the pain they're feeling or will feel if they don't do as you suggest. Since we constantly try to distract ourselves from pain, stirring up another's pain isn't a mean thing to do. Rather, it can be a positive step in helping a person to change. For example, if you wanted to sell someone a health club membership, showing beautiful people having a great time would likely stir up an overweight person's pain. Once they felt this, you could more easily get them to enroll in your new health club. Both you and they would benefit.

3) Ask effective questions. The best questions to ask are those that help stir up someone's pain (as a precondition to being a motivated "buyer"), or questions to find out a person's

needs or values. Below I have several questions in each of these two categories:

Pain-Inducing Questions:

1. What would happen if.... (provide a worst case scenario, such as "you didn't lose your extra weight and you had a health problem as a result")?

2. What bothers you about (fill in the blank of a competing product or service)?

3. If you keep doing/buying _____, what might you miss out on?

4. How might your life be better if you no longer had this problem? (Of course, your product or service aims to overcome this problem.)

The advantage of asking pain-inducing questions is that it allows the person to whom you're "selling" to sell themselves on your idea or product. They're much more likely to believe their own statements than yours. Once they're in touch with the possible pain they'll experience by not following your advice, they'll be much more open to your idea or product.

Needs and Values Questions:

1. What do you most like about (their current way of doing things)?

2. What do you look for in a... (whatever you're offering them)?

3. What's most important to you when considering buying a...?

4. How will you know when it's time to change to a new...?

5. What do you see as a major problem you (or your company) are having right now?

6. What needs to happen for us to more forward with ...?

As you can see, the questions in this second category help you to more precisely know exactly what someone needs and desires. Once you know this information, all you need to do is show how your product or service can help them out. Of course, if what you have to sell doesn't meet their current needs, tell them. In this way, you'll create even more trust, which may be useful at some later date.

4) Invite people into the pleasure they'll feel by following your suggestions. Once people are in touch with their pain, they want to know that there is a simple way out. By painting a mental picture of the benefits they'll receive from buying what you're selling, you'll have the power of both pain and pleasure working for you. You can use simple phrases to help people imagine their desired outcome. For instance, you might say, "Think of how relaxing it would be if...." or "Imagine how much better you'd feel knowing that...." or "Soon, you could be enjoying...." When creating a mental picture for someone else, it's best to use specific, emotional images and words. To say "This fast car is made really well and is very safe to drive" does not inspire most people. Contrast that with this statement: "This screaming turbo-

charged engine is made as precisely as a Rolex watch, and is as safe as an armored tank!" Hopefully, you can sense the difference.

Like most skills, the ability to persuade people is gained by having the right methods, concepts, and distinctions. Once you know the basics, you can always learn the more subtle ideas and methods. Yet most mastery in life comes from simply practicing the fundamentals, and there are no shortcuts for practicing. Believe me, I've tried. By knowing how to get rapport, memorizing some of the questions listed previously, understanding the importance of stirring up someone's pain, and by knowing how to get people to imagine the pleasure of your idea or product, you'll notice a major difference in how effectively you sell. There is no substitute for sincerity, however. You must really believe that whatever you're selling, from a widget to an early bedtime for your son, really is in their best interest. So refrain from selling things you don't believe in. That will allow you to sell with integrity, and as you practice "helping" people rather than "selling" to them, you'll find that everyone will benefit.

39: Market Yourself to Riches

Integrity Marketing Principles

When people come across the word *marketing,* they rarely get excited. Yet by understanding the five principles of what I call "integrity marketing," you can make your dreams come true—and have a great time doing it.

1) Market something you truly believe in. To passionately believe in something, it is necessary to know that what you're marketing will strongly benefit people. The more you know this, the easier it is to be fully passionate about it. When you are convinced that your product or service will be of much greater benefit to your "customers" than the price they will have to pay, you have taken the most important step toward successful marketing. For example, most of us would have a hard time marketing a seminar that lacked any really useful information. Yet it would be easy to market a seminar that *guaranteed* to help people make an extra $5,000 in income in just one month if you *really* believed it could deliver the goods.

2) Be willing to find out what others truly want, and to become committed to providing it for them. We've all heard the business maxim, "Find a need and fill it." When you can meet someone's need and pursue your passion at the same time, then you really have a powerful combination. Since I feel passionate about meditation, I figured I would try to come up with a meditation tape that people would really love. Before I created the tape I asked dozens of people why they didn't regularly meditate. I learned that most people don't meditate regularly because they feel they don't have enough time, or they find it too boring. Therefore, I became committed to making a short tape that would give people an immediate and profound experience. I finally created *The Ten-Minute Pure Love Meditation Experience,* and it's now one of my bestselling products.

3) Recognize the value of people and find ways to make them want to work with you or be your customer. Whatever your financial, personal, or spiritual dreams, they can't be fulfilled

without truly caring for people. If you own a store, your job is to make people feel good about doing business with you. Besides offering them products or services that are helpful, you can make them feel valued in other ways. Just as in intimate relationships, little things can make a big difference in how much people feel valued. A nice smile, a kind word, or simply a sincere desire to be of help can go a long way in making your business stand out above the rest.

I used to go to a copy shop that was near where I lived, but the attitude of the employees toward the customers was always very poor. Although it was a bit out of my way, one day I decided to go to another copy shop. The owner greeted me with a warm smile, as if he were really happy to see me. I told him what I needed copied and asked him when I could pick it up. To my surprise he said, "I'll do it right now—it'll only take a few minutes." As he copied my material, he began a friendly conversation with me and seemed truly interested in what I was writing. As I paid for the copies, he asked me if I would like some free memo pads to use as scrap paper. Indeed, I needed some memo pads, and he gave me about a dozen of them. He asked me if I wanted a box or help carrying the stuff out to my car. I felt that I was being treated like royalty. He made a customer for life.

In business, there's an obscure term called "the marginal net worth per customer." In essence, this term refers to the amount of money you stand to make from a single customer over the life of your business. To figure this out accurately, you need to also include the amount of money you might receive from all the referred business you receive from a given customer. In the case of me and the copy shop, I once figured that I have spent about $1,200 a year at this friendly man's copy shop, of which about $1,000 ends up being his profit. Over the last seven years, that means he's made roughly $7,000 profit from me. But the story doesn't end there. I've told at least twenty people about this copy shop, and about half of them have become his loyal customers. If they spend the same amount as I do, that means he's ultimately made $70,000 from having me as a customer over the past seven years! That's a nice reward for just a few minutes of good service.

How much is each customer worth to you? Do you treat the people you do business with like they were worth a million dollars, or like they're just ordinary customers? Figuring out the marginal net worth of each customer you do business with can be an eye-opening experience. It can help you see that each highly satisfied patron can have a major impact on your financial life. Remember, customers know when you're just being courteous to make an extra buck, and when you're being helpful because you really care about people. It's nice to know that purity of heart can result in more business and money.

4) Understand the potential power of commitment. If you have a dream that you really believe in, then you need to be willing to persevere until it becomes a reality. As I've come to know many successful authors and entrepreneurs, I've seen that all of them share the trait of being fully committed to whatever they are marketing. It's almost as if they won't take no for an answer. It's not that they're pushy, they just believe so much in what they're doing that they persist despite the many trials they inevitably encounter.

5) Learn to use your intuition as the basis for making important business decisions. Despite the fact that knowledge and expertise are helpful in any business, no one can consistently state what will do well and what won't. Therefore, successful business people are not afraid to use their intuition as an aid in making important decisions. They know that intuition, hunches, and gut feelings can sometimes be more important than market research, past experience, or rational analysis.

A study was done several years ago in which two groups of executives were given ESP tests. The first group of executives had businesses that were doing particularly well. They were highly regarded in their fields because they seemed to make a lot of the right moves in their businesses. The second group of executives had businesses in a slump. While being at the top of their company, they had made decisions that led to poorer sales and profits in their businesses. When these two groups were given ESP tests, they found that the successful executives scored 500 percent better at ESP abilities than their less successful counterparts. The conclusion the authors of this study made was that successful business people use psychic abilities without even knowing it, and are therefore more successful.

In the world of business, we are constantly faced with decisions. What product should we sell, what ad should we run, what service should we focus on? Gathering as much information as possible is necessary to the success of any business. Yet, as multifaceted beings, we need to respect both the analytical and intuitive sides of our nature. By gathering rational information *and* listening to the "still, small voice" within, we can improve our chances of success. As one becomes better at applying the principles of integrity marketing, it's possible to do a lot of honorable work in the world—and have a good time doing it.

40: Experience Greater Abundance

Tapping into the Power of Generosity

Science has progressed rapidly over the last hundred years because it uses experiments to verify or disprove certain principles. In a similar way, you and I can test things out in order to learn valuable ways of experiencing greater abundance. What I'm going to suggest here is that you try tithing (giving away 10 percent of your income) for a predetermined period of time in order to see what effect it has on your personal and/or financial life. As in any scientific procedure, when doing a tithing experiment, you'd get the most benefit if you carefully noticed the results of your new behavior. If you noticed that over a six-month period of tithing your income dramatically increased, you felt more loving, and you felt better about yourself, then you could say your experiment indicated that tithing "works" for you. On the other hand, if you noticed tithing led to even more anxiety about money, then you'd be smart to try a different way to contribute to others. Still, I believe tithing works, and I urge you to try it.

Experiments can help people learn new things and try new behaviors they might never try otherwise. It's a lot less frightening to try tithing for a single month than it is to decide to tithe for the rest of your life. If your month-long trial run proved promising, it wouldn't be very hard to try a long-term tithing commitment. When it comes to finances, most people are hesitant to put their money where their heart is. They play the money game strictly by the rules of logic, rather than by spiritual principles. By conducting short-term money experiments, we can gradually become free of our prison of rationality. When our tests are "successful"—meaning they lead to more peace, money, or contribution—we expand. When our efforts lead to less peace, money, or contribution, we learn valuable lessons.

The first thing I did during my initial month-long experiment of tithing was buy about $25 worth of ice cream and go to the local beach with a sign that read "Free Ice Cream." Finally, as my ice cream began to melt, a cute little six-year old girl walked up and asked me in a shy voice, "How much is your free ice cream?" I told her that if she gave me a smile, I'd give her a double scoop for nothing. She squealed with delight. When watchful parents saw that the little girl didn't die from food poisoning, the mass pilgrimage to my holy ice cream stand began.

As I scooped up smile after smile for wide-eyed kids, many suspicious parents began asking me why I was giving away free ice cream. I told them, "I like to do nice things for people because it makes me feel good." That seemed to satisfy their suspicion. As I scooped up ice cream for their kids, several of the parents asked me what I did for a living. I told them I was a psychotherapist. Four people asked me for my business card. Since I was at the beach to give away ice cream, I didn't have my card, but I told them my number was in the phone book. Three of the people I met that day actually did call for appointments. Months later I added up all the money I made from the appointments I had with these three people, and it totaled over $1,000. That's a pretty good reward for having a good time, making a lot of people happy, and spending only $25 on ice cream!

After a month of randomly doing kind things for people, I realized I felt better about myself. I was also making more money due to business I picked up from treating people with more kindness and respect. Therefore, I decided to be kind to strangers as a way of life. By writing in my journal periodically throughout my initial "kindness experiment," I had proof that acting this way was beneficial to me (as well as others). Seeing this effect inspired me to look into the possibility of giving away 10 percent of my income. Although I had read that tithing can be a very beneficial practice, I was always too cheap to try it out. Still, the success of my kindness experiment suggested I might be able to find a way to tithe that did not overwhelm me.

Traditionally, tithing has been the practice of giving away 10 percent of one's income to a religious organization, such as a church or synagogue. I felt that this was too impersonal for me, so I wanted to try "tithing" in a way that helped me feel less worried about money and more generous with the people I feel closest to. After trying various methods, I came upon a formula that has worked quite well. In essence, I've decided that 10 percent of what I make is not my personal money, but "God's money." I have a separate account for this money, and once a month, I spend time getting quiet inside and ask for guidance about who or where this money should go. I often get a clear intuitive sense of where "God's money" should go, and how much should go there. Since this money is in a different account and is not really "mine," it's easy to surrender control and simply listen for what would be best to do with it. If I don't receive a clear message, I just allow the money to sit in the account until the next time I ask.

I sometimes ask my intuition if I can dip into the "God's money" account for a purpose that benefits me. For example, recently I had several clients who didn't pay me, and I was feeling resentful, hurt, and anxious. In a moment of quiet meditation, I asked if it was okay to receive the money I was owed from my tithing account. The answer I received was "yes." Receiving this money from my tithing account helped me feel at peace. I quickly let go of the anger I'd been feeling toward the clients who hadn't paid me. Previously, I used to be greatly bothered by clients who didn't pay me, or when I had things stolen.

While doing this loose form of tithing may seem less than ideal, it has allowed me to consistently give to others while avoiding becoming anxious about money. Since I now know that 10 percent of the money I make isn't "mine," I feel more at ease at giving money away to worthy people and causes. It's resulted in a freer, more relaxed feeling about money. It has also led me to being more generous with people. Once each month I ask "How can I use this money to bring more joy and healing into the world?" I receive different answers each time I ask. Sometimes I'll feel a desire to give money to a friend in need, or a gift they'll appreciate. Other times I'll write a check to a charity that I feel does important work. Because I am not writing a check from "my" account, I can better give this money away with a true feeling of service. If this way of tithing seems like it might work for you, I suggest you try it as an experiment and see how it feels. It could change how abundant you feel, as well as how relaxed you are about giving to yourself and others.

41: Program Your Subconscious For Success

Self-Hypnosis Made Easy

When I was twelve, my uncle managed to transform my normally shy sister into Mick Jagger. As she belted out a pretty good rendition of "Satisfaction" in front of my family, I was impressed. With five minutes of gentle talking, my uncle had hypnotized my sister into thinking she was an entirely different person. After seeing this demonstration, I thought that perhaps hypnosis could help me change how I felt about myself, which at the time was not very good. I started reading books on hypnosis, and applying it every day. I soon noticed that how I felt about myself began to improve in dramatic ways, and my life got better too. I learned that by "reprogramming" certain beliefs in the subconscious mind, a person could quickly change specific aspects of their behavior. Fortunately, to hypnotize yourself does not require years of instruction. In fact, it's easy, safe, and effective. By following the steps I suggest, you can change some of your subconscious beliefs about yourself, and thereby increase your level of success.

Why hypnosis? The human mind is like an iceberg. What is visible, the conscious mind, is only a very small portion of what is going on. Ninety percent of the mind is subconscious. While not consciously apparent to us, the subconscious is continually affecting our behavior and perceptions. To put in new "programming" into the subconscious requires at least one of three things: repetition, deep relaxation, or emotional intensity. Repetition is useful because whatever the conscious mind thinks of enough, the subconscious will eventually accept.

Deep relaxation is useful because when we're deeply relaxed, the normal defenses we have to accepting new information are temporarily put aside. Finally, emotional intensity is helpful for reaching the subconscious. When words or images are powerful enough, they tend to impact us on a subconscious level. By using the principles of repetition, deep relaxation, and emotional intensity when hypnotizing yourself, new programming can be "wired" into your subconscious.

About a decade ago, I had no money. I realized that a major reason for this was my subconscious blocks to success. While on a conscious level I wanted money, subconsciously I equated money with greed, busyness, worry, and problems. No wonder I never had any! Using self-hypnosis I hypnotized myself to change my subconscious associations to wealth. Within five years I had enough money to travel around the world for six months, buy a house, and put a lot of money into savings.

In order to hypnotize yourself, it'll help if you have a cassette recorder of some kind. If you don't have one, you can now buy one for about $25. The easiest way to hypnotize yourself is to listen to a tape of yourself going through the "trance-inducing" process. At its core, hypnosis is a very simple skill to learn. In fact, I have provided a transcript for you to record into the tape player to hypnotize yourself. It's important that you read this transcript very slowly, and in somewhat of a monotone voice. Part I of the transcript should take about eight to ten minutes to complete. Part II of the hypnotic process is where you put in the new programming you desire. For your convenience, I've included the suggestions I used for myself in changing how I felt about wealth and my ability to manifest greater success. Of course, you may choose to reprogram other ideas or suggestions into your subconscious. That's okay. Just be sure to write it down and, at the appropriate time, speak it slowly into the cassette recorder.

The third and final part of the hypnotic process is the "awakening" phase. Actually, in hypnosis, people don't fall asleep. In fact, you'll be very aware of everything you hear on the tape. You'll just feel extremely relaxed and may think that nothing is happening. The combination of relaxation, repetition, and powerful images allows your words to reach the subconscious mind. Since the subconscious mind controls most of our behavior, the impact of your words will be much larger than if you heard the same words in a normal state of mind. If you record this transcript into a tape player, it should take between twelve and twenty minutes, especially if you say it very slowly, and at each "pause" in parentheses you are silent for about ten seconds. Remember to read this at a very, very, very slow pace when recording it into your cassette recorder:

Part I—The Induction Phase

Find a comfortable place to sit or lie down, and take a deep, slow breath. (pause) Feel your right foot. Notice any tension in your foot, and allow it to relax. (pause) Now notice how your left foot feels. Once again, allow your foot to completely relax. (pause) Gradually, you can begin to feel your lower legs, your calf muscles, let go of any tension. With each breath that you breathe, you feel your legs relax more and more. Now you can feel your upper legs become as relaxed and at ease as your lower legs. With each word you hear, and each breath you breathe, your legs become even more relaxed. (pause) Now become aware of your right hand. Allow it to relax, as if you could feel it being soothed in a warm pool of energy. Allow this feeling of relaxation to move into your right forearm, and finally your right upper arm. Feel the muscles in your right arm become loose and limp. Good. Now become aware of your left arm and hand. Feel your left hand and arm become as relaxed as your right, from the tips of your fingers all the way up to the top of your arm. (pause)

With each breath that you take, imagine breathing in a favorite color of soothing, nurturing air deep into your lungs. With each exhalation, imagine breathing out any remaining stress or tension that was in your body. Breathing in soothing, relaxing air, exhaling tension and stress. (pause) Now become aware of the muscles in your face—your jaw, cheeks, and forehead muscles. Allow them to melt into complete relaxation. Good. Imagine yourself at the top of a set of stairs, and as I count backwards from ten to zero, picture yourself walking down the stairs to a deeper level of relaxation and a deeper level of mind. Ten. (pause) Nine, eight, imagining yourself going down to a deeper level of relaxation. Seven, six. You become open to new learning, behavior and sensations as you take a step down to five. Four, three, deeper and deeper, two, one, and now zero. Deeply relaxed and open to new learning.

Part II—The Reprogramming Phase

You can create your own suggestions for this part, but below is a sample of suggestions to be more open to financial and personal success:

Think back to a time when you felt fully abundant; it may have been a long time ago or recently. It may have been a day with friends, in nature, or after a big success in your career.

(pause) Try to remember what was happening and how good it felt to feel prosperous, secure, and confident. Imagine that with each breath you breathe in, you could literally expand and enhance the feeling of abundance you feel. (pause) With this feeling of success, and the right resources, you could accomplish whatever dreams you wish to achieve. Imagine feeling grateful and excited about how your career and finances are going. Picture yourself taking the next positive step forward in your job. See yourself succeeding and feeling excited by all the good fortune you're experiencing. Imagine taking the extra money you now have and using it to help friends, family, and to pursue your own personal dreams of travel, a beautiful place to live, or whatever you most desire. (pause) As you express your gifts in the world and create financial and personal success, consider how good it feels to be living so fully and passionately. Enjoy the feeling of being proud of who you are and what you've accomplished. (pause) Know that, as you focus on who you want to be and what you want to create, your subconscious automatically pulls you in that direction. With each day, you find yourself taking the small actions necessary to insure long-lasting personal and financial success.

Part III—The Awakening Phase

I am now going to gradually count to ten. As I count from one to ten, you can imagine yourself walking up the stairs to greater wakefulness. One, two, feel your legs starting to return back to a normal feeling. Three, four, five, your arms and body beginning to feel like they're waking up from a refreshing sleep. Six, seven, feeling good, better than you've felt in a long time. Eight, getting ready to stretch and open your eyes. Nine, feeling awake, and ten, open your eyes and enjoy your day.

Once you've recorded this on tape, simply play it back in a room where you will not be distracted. The more you can picture and feel yourself being successful, the more effective this tape will be in helping you move in the direction of your goals. If you desire, feel free to add your own suggestions to Part II of the tape, or even write entirely different suggestions that fit your personal goals. Listening to a tape such as this is especially powerful upon arising in the morning or right before going to bed at night. Whenever you listen to it, you'll find it a powerful tool in assisting you in achieving the success you desire.

Last, but Not Least:

It's always easier to read about ideas and methods than it is to use them. Fortunately, in this book there are a lot of ideas and tools that are incredibly easy to use. If you haven't already done so, choose one or two methods that particularly interest you and begin using them *now*. Because these tools are so effective in changing people's lives, there is a subtle form of resistance to using them. For various reasons, our subconscious mind is afraid of change and therefore part of you will likely resist applying these methods in your daily life. If you can overcome your initial resistance, you'll find that the changes you create as you use this information will bring you more harmony, health, and happiness.

Success is not a destination. It is a journey of continual growth and movement toward becoming a better, more capable, harmonious, and loving person. One of the best ways to accelerate your growth is to surround yourself with like-minded people who are also interested in becoming better human beings. By having a group of friends who are committed to personal development, you'll have an increased chance of keeping true to your higher ideals and aspirations. I encourage you to seek out such people if they are not already in your life. If you already have friends focused on personal growth, I hope you'll share with them the ideas you've found valuable from this book. On our own, we can do little, but with the help and accountability of friends it is much easier to keep our heart open and our dreams alive. As you practice these tools, my hope is that you'll use your increasing level of success to help those who are less fortunate than yourself.

Acknowledgments

I first want to acknowledge the various folks at Conari Press for being a pleasure to work with. I especially want to thank Claudia Schaab, Nina Lesowitz, Brenda Knight, and Mary Jane Ryan. Many of the tools in this book were made popular or originated from other people. In that regard I want to thank Frank Sanitate (time-management suggestions), Helena Kay (health information), Tony Robbins, Simon D'Arcy, Edward de Bono, and Steve Foss (for health-related information.) I also want to thank Kirsten Young for supporting me in life and at my workshops, and my mother for helping me to market my books. (It's definitely helpful to have a Jewish mother when you're an author.) Finally, my ability to write books about personal growth and success wouldn't be possible without my long association with my teacher, mentor, and planetary guide, Justin Gold. Thank you all.

About the Author

Jonathan Robinson is an author, professional speaker, and psychotherapist who lives in Santa Barbara, California. Through his company, *Tools for Success,* he specializes in teaching individuals, businesses, and associations practical and powerful ways to increase their level of personal and business success. He has written six other books, including *Communication Miracles for Couples, Shortcuts to Bliss,* and *The Little Book of Big Questions.* Mr. Robinson is a frequent guest on shows such as *Oprah, Geraldo,* and *CNN,* and his work has been featured in *USA Today, Newsweek,* and dozens of other publications.

Mr. Robinson conducts keynote talks and seminars for businesses interested in increasing their level of productivity, motivation, and profits. Three of his most requested talks are:

1. The Power to Live Your Dreams and Achieve Your Goals

2. Mastering the One-Minute Relationship (for sales)

3. Communication Magic: How to Solve Problems Without Bruising Egos

If you would like information about his talks, or if you would like a free copy of his catalog of audio tapes and book titles, please contact him at: www.howtotools.com or

OR e-mail him at: Iamjonr@aol.com

OR Fax: (805) 967-4128

OR Write: Jonathan Robinson
              278 Via El Encantador
              Santa Barbara, CA 93111

CONARI PRESS, established in 1987, publishes books on topics ranging from psychology, spirituality, and women's history to sexuality, parenting, and personal growth. Our main goal is to publish quality books that will make a difference in people's lives—both how we feel about ourselves and how we relate to one another.

Our readers are our most important resource, and we value your input, suggestions, and ideas. We'd love to hear from you—after all, we are publishing books for you!

To request our latest book catalog or to be added to our mailing list, please contact:

CONARI PRESS
2550 Ninth Street, Suite 101
Berkeley, California 94710-2551
800-685-9595   510-649-7175
fax: 510-649-7190   e-mail: conari@conari.com
www.conari.com